MW01246016

Diet and Exercise for Women Over 50

Reset your diet and exercise if you are a woman after 50 with a plant-based diet meal plan

© Copyright - All rights reserved.

The content contained within this book may not be reproduced, duplicated, or transmitted without direct written permission from the author or the publisher.

Under no circumstances will any blame or legal responsibility be held against the publisher, or author, for any damages, reparation, or monetary loss due to the information contained within this book. Either directly or indirectly.

Legal Notice:

This book is copyright protected. This book is only for personal use. You cannot amend, distribute, sell, use, quote, or paraphrase any part, or the content within this book, without the consent of the author or publisher.

Disclaimer Notice:

Please note the information contained within this document is for educational and entertainment purposes only. All effort has been executed to present accurate, up to date, and reliable, complete information. No warranties of any kind are declared or implied. Readers acknowledge that the author is not engaging in the rendering of legal, financial, medical, or professional advice. The content within this book has been derived from various sources. Please consult a licensed professional before attempting any techniques outlined in this book.

By reading this document, the reader agrees that under no circumstances is the author responsible for any losses, direct or indirect, which are incurred as a result of the use of the information contained within this document, including, but not limited to, — errors, omissions, or inaccuracies.

Description

Thinking about adopting a plant-based diet? The information you need is outlined to make fantastic changes to your lifestyle that will improve your health, your skin, your digestion, and even your joint health. Don't delay in making changes to your life. Plant-based diets are becoming more and more common. It is not a fad. It is a sustainable change to the way you live that makes real improvements in the way you live and how you feel daily.

Reduce inflammation in your joints and tendons.

Lose weight and offset the unwelcome changes in your body from menopause.

Learn about the advantages of organic products and why they are necessary to eat clean.

Learn about eating whole foods to feel full while consuming flavorful and delicious foods that you create on your own.

Take advantage of the variety of produce available in most markets. You feel like you are traveling the globe with cuisine from different parts of the world that are being grown locally.

Combine the best ingredients with the best nutritional value to make the changes to your plant-based lifestyle worth the effort.

Learn which foods to avoid eating to make it easy to eat clean, whole foods.

Not sure how to adjust to exercising with your new middle-aged body, look no further. The answers are here.

Get motivated to change your diet and expand your capabilities to exercise.

Make the changes today with the tools listed here.

Growing old is not always easy. Get the information you need to transform your life with diet and exercise. Learn the advantages of adopting a plant-based diet, even after the age of 50. Learn how menopause affects your body and why this diet will help with symptoms of menopause. Learn how you can determine how many calories you should be eating each day. Figure out your body mass index and determine whether it is in an acceptable range for the average person of your age and gender. Gain the tools to see what markers of physical fitness you have already achieved and where you may need to work a little harder. Combine diet and exercise to extend your life and make your life easier to live. This diet and exercise have the power to recharge your life. You will have tools to reverse some of the negative health aspects of your body and positively impact your health. Use the diet to proactively improve your heart health, reduce bad cholesterol, and increase good cholesterol levels. Adopt a diet that may defend your body against some types of cancer. Lose fat and develop more muscle. This isn't about vanity; it's about healthy living. You will feel better, look better, and improve brain function by using the instruction outlined in this book. Food and exercise matter a great deal in how you feel. By improving your health, you will find that you feel better about your life and yourself. Take control of your life by controlling your diet.

Table of contents

Introduction

Congratulations on purchasing *Diet and Exercise for Women Over 50* and thank you for doing so.

This book is for women over the age of 50 who want to know how to kickstart their life with a plant-based diet and exercise. You will learn why you have been gaining weight and what you can do to combat the hormone changes occurring and making your muscle mass a shadow of what it was previously. Learn how to focus your energies on being healthy and doing things you enjoy, all while improving the quality of your life. The best way to improve your life, as you enter your golden years, is through healthy eating and moderate exercise. Learn the key factors in improving yourself by strengthening your bones and increasing muscle. Fit the facts in the book into your lifestyle to recapture the vigor of your past life and ease out of menopause without gaining weight.

There are plenty of books on this subject on the market, thanks again for choosing this one! Every effort was made to ensure it is full of as much useful information as possible, please enjoy it!

Chapter 1: Why Do You Need a Reset

As women age, lifestyle, and diet matter more than ever before. For most women, by the time they reach the age of 50, it becomes necessary to make adjustments, be them large or small, to do away with old habits and make changes necessary to create a healthy body and spirit. Food that was previously a diet staple can suddenly make life miserable by suddenly turning on you, making you feel uncomfortable if not unwell. By taking control of your life and taking measures to counteract the negative effects of growing old, it will be possible to maximize positive health potential by eating organic food with a plant-based foundation.

Why do we call it a reset? It is going to be a new start for your body. By starting with food, the fuel of your body, you will be able to cleanse the toxins from your organs and detoxify your body to promote a new healthy physical environment. This will be important for you as you begin to tackle two major issues for women over the age of fifty, weight control and bone and joint health.

Weight Control

One of the first things you may notice as you enter post-menopausal life is that clothes are fitting tighter, and the numbers are creeping higher on the scale. Unfortunately, the metabolism slows as we age. This means that eating the same number of calories that you have always consumed can add pounds. The slower metabolism causes calories to be burned at a slower rate. The only way to gain weight if for the number of calories consumed to exceed the number of calories burned as fuel. The body is burning calories even when we are not doing anything. This rate slows down as we get older. If you don't adjust your caloric intake to match the reduction in calories burned, the excess calories start to turn into pounds. After having your thyroid checked, if everything is fine, you will want to make the changes necessary to match your calorie intake to your new metabolism. This is one of the reasons why you may need to look at what you're eating when you're eating at and how much of it, you're eating. It's simply a normal reaction to your body as you grow older.

the way that fat is distributed around your body also changes as you age. Unfortunately, that tends to accumulate around your waist, which can lead to high blood pressure and heart disease. This makes it important to modify your caloric intake to minimize weight gain and work towards preventing obesity as you grow older. Many times, obesity and excess weight are directly related to poor nutritional habits. When you rely on a diet that's high in sugar and salt, your body starts to build up resistance to insulin wish may trigger inflammatory diseases like dementia and type 2 diabetes. one of the easiest things to do to modify your diet is to simply start cutting out things that you know are not nutritional and do not provide value to your diet. If you add foods to your diet that have high nutritional value is like fresh fruits and vegetables, nuts, and seeds, you will find that you'll be able to fill up unhealthy foods and eliminate some of the ways to calories and your diet.

It is important to add calories to your diet that are healthy for you. Keeping in mind that 3500 calories are a pound, you need to determine how many calories you need based on your actual lifestyle and how your body is utilizing food that you're eating. Since the early muscle mass may be decreasing, you want to make sure that the muscle mass is not being replaced by fat. You may find that you need to reduce the amount of fat that you are consuming. You may also need to change the type of pets that you're eating to those that are more easily digested. Changes in your body structure make it necessary to reduce the calories that you are consuming, and you may need to adjust this type of calories that you're eating. Even if you are consistently eating the same foods that you've always eaten, your body may not be able to digest increase sensitivity to food items and a breakdown of some of the internal functions of your body. If you are not careful, you can easily and 50 lb. to your weight within 5 to 10 years. Because it is more difficult to lose weight as you age, it is important to modify your food consumption so that you're not possibly gaining weight over time.

What is a Healthy Weight?

To determine what a healthy weight is for you, you will have to calculate your BMI is your body mass index. This calculation gives an estimate of the average weight that is healthy for your height. You can generally find a BMI calculator on the internet but here's the formula for your BMI:

$703*weight$ (in lbs.)/height (in inches) ^{2}

So, if you are a 5'5inch woman weighing 160lbs, your BMI is calculated by multiplying 703 * 160, which equals 112480 lbs. Then you check the height in inches squared so that's 65 inches squared are 4225 inches. And you divide 112485 by 4225. The result is a BMI of 26.62 lbs./inch.

Normal BMI is usually between 18.5 and 24.9 for women. As you can see, a BMI of 26.62 is above the range that would be considered healthy and most women. This indicates that there should be an effort made to lose weight. Because we can easily gain weight, you can see how it is important to work to maintain a healthy BMI. This is often done through diet. For women over 50, minimum caloric intake is generally around 1600 calories per day. This would be for a person who does not participate in any physical activities and has a relatively sedentary lifestyle. People who participate in moderate activities like yard work, walking swiftly, stretching, hiking, and easy bike rides can generally increase their calorie intake to eat 1800 calories a day. People who are very active and Hutchinson pain in my swimming, weight lifting, riding a bicycle at greater than 10 miles per hour walking at more than 4 miles per hour will usually need to increase their calorie intake throughout to 2,000 calories per day.

That is a lot of activity for someone who may have a limited range of flexibility and stamina. Fortunately, you can work up to these levels of activity over time. The amount of food you eat or vary depending on the calorie count and portion size of food that you're choosing. It may be necessary to modify what you're eating to be able to feel full, especially if you are expending a lot of calories through physical activity. physical activity will help to build muscle mass and maintain the mass that you already have. Read labels to determine the portion size and nutritional value for what you're eating.

In reality, you may not need as many calories to be healthy as you age. Many people have lifestyles that are slowing down. Even if you're just as active as you were previously, your body organs are not as new and fresh as they used to be, and they need to be nourished in different ways. One of these ways is that there is not a need for the same number of calories to be consumed to be considered as having a healthy diet. All things being equal, the number of calories that you need will not be as great as when you were younger. consider it as your body's organs becoming more efficient as they age. The excess calories tend to present themselves as punches to the belly and additional way in the thighs and hips a woman. This is a minor weight gain for people of average weight before menopause. For people who were heavier before the changes in hormones, the problem is usually exacerbated, and the increases are greater. It is a good idea to make adjustments and provide fuel for your body and limit the number of excess calories and fats that may have provided comfort over the years.

Joint and Bone Health

As women age, the risk of osteoporosis increases. Calcium is not produced by the body and must be consumed as part of a balanced diet. The daily recommended dosage of calcium for women over 50 is 1200 milligrams per day. This high amount of calcium is necessary to prevent osteoporosis and other bone-related issues. Because the ability of the body to absorb calcium decreases as women age, it is important to increase the amount of calcium consumed. Coupled with the decreased ability to absorb calcium, it is also more difficult for many women to digest dairy products, which is what many people rely upon as a source of calcium. Fortunately, calcium can also be found in dark green leafy vegetables and calcium-fortified beverages like orange juice.

Since up to one-third of women over the age of fifty are at risk of breaking a bone due to the effects of osteoporosis, women need to eat an appropriate amount of calcium-rich foods each day. The absorption rate of calcium increases if vitamin D is also introduced with the calcium. Many times, it is recommended that dietary supplements are included in the diet to be sure adequate amounts of calcium are consumed. Often, this is achieved by eating foods rich in calcium and taking a vitamin D supplement to help the calcium absorb into the bones, thereby strengthening the bones of the body. Supplements should be considered a last resort; the food sources of calcium and vitamin D are more easily tolerated by the body and more effective forms of nourishment. Foods rich in calcium include:

Dairy products like milk, cheese, and yogurt. Nutritional labels for these products provide the information needed to know how much calcium is included per serving. One cup (8 oz) of milk has over 300 mg of calcium, 1 ounce of cheese has around 200 mg of calcium, and yogurt has 250 mg of calcium in an 8 oz serving.

Dark green leafy vegetables like collard greens and kale have a large amount of calcium. One cup of cooked green leafy vegetables has approximately 250 mg of calcium. Spinach is also high in calcium, but it contains a chemical makeup that makes it difficult for the body to absorb its calcium, so it is not as good a choice as a food to eat for its calcium value.

Bone Density Changes

The changes in bone density can be chalked up to a few factors. One factor is that over time the bones structure breaks down as any hard surface will after years and years of use. After menopause, estrogen levels are very low. Estrogen is the hormone that protects bones in women. This, coupled with the fact that women tend to have thinner bones than men, creates a situation that causes the bone mass to deteriorate after estrogen is no longer produced as a result of menopause. With estrogen no longer protecting the bones, a large percentage of the mask and decrease within five to seven years of menopause. Many women are also lactose intolerant and avoid consumption of dairy products, which are high in calcium. This is especially true among African-American and Asian-American women. The decrease levels of estrogen and the continuing decrease in bone mass cause many women to be prone to hip fractures. Many women have decreased bone density even though they do not suffer from osteoporosis. The issues of bone mass need to be addressed to continue a healthy lifestyle. Diet can certainly be changed to increase calcium consumption and absorption. Exercise will also be a factor.

Exercise is important in maintain and strengthen your body. This includes strong bones and muscles. Over the age of 50, women may not have the desire or be able to perform some of the exercises that combat muscle loss such as jumping. what is recommended for women over 50 is an increase in resistance training. these are exercises and activities that build muscle that is attached to the bone and will, as a result, increase bone density and grow bong. These include exercises like weight training and running, particularly on stairs. high impact aerobics is also a good exercise for increasing bone density in older women.

Slower Metabolism

One of the primary causes of weight gain for women over the age of 50 is the result of a reduced amount of estrogen in the bloodstream. Metabolism is the body's process for converting food and beverages to energy. This energy is used during periods of activity and helps the body store energy when your body is at rest. When the body is resting, the hormone levels in the body rejuvenate and assist with energy storage and the overall efficiencies of the body.

Slows with Aging

The metabolism slows with a j because it is a normal function of the body. In women over 50, levels of estrogen are decreased and affect the metabolic rate of the body. Estrogen is known to regulate metabolism in the body. After menopause, there is less estrogen in the body, and they rid of potassium slows dramatically. Because the rate of metabolism slows, your body will have less energy and you will be less inclined to exercise. because the ovaries are producing less estrogen, particularly estradiol. Estradiol helps to regulate body weight and as levels decrease in the body, there is a tendency to gain weight. the lower amounts of estrogen in the system may also be responsible for increased amounts of fat in the stomach area and around organs. When fat is surrounding various organs, this leads to catastrophic diseases like diabetes, heart disease, and stroke.

After menopause is complete, metabolism typically slows in women. This causes decreased energy as well as weight gain. The fact that a slower metabolism occurs after menopause is because of the reduced levels of estrogen. Estrogen helps insulin process food and assisting weight loss. Estrogen also helps women maintain muscle mass. With the lack of this chemical hormone in the body, a cookies weight gain and loss of muscle must be combated through diet and exercise.

Metabolism is the process of breaking down fats into energy. When the energy is transformed from the proteins in the body, efficient use of what you eat results. For this reason, when estrogen is no longer being produced in the ovaries, there is the difficulty of maintaining weight levels based on your historical consumption of the same a lot of calories.

Food Choices Make a Difference

After the age of 50, with the reduction of estrogen affecting the rate of metabolism, you may want to boost your metabolism by heating foods well help make up the difference. One thing that your diet will appreciate is protein. The rate of protein consumption should be monitored so that you're not consuming more calories than you will expend in a day. Plant-based proteins are very effective in assisting to increase your metabolism.

One of the most effective ways of introducing plant-based protein into your diet is to make sure you're consuming grains that are high in protein. Some examples of these grains are amaranth, which was 9 grams of protein per cup, and chickpeas which I have 14 grams of protein per cup. Nuts and seeds are also common sources of protein when you are following a meatless diet. Many nuts are high in fat so you have to be sure to eat low-fat options of nut proteins.

If you have previously relied on animal protein to fulfill your dietary needs, you may find that you need additional amino acids to promote the transition of protein to energy. This will require a good mix of plant proteins to be sure that the proteins are absorbed into your system at an adequate rate. Also, if you are going to rely on non-processed plant proteins, you must be sure that your diet is well-rounded to consume vitamins and nutrients to sustain the body, your metabolism and be positively affected by drinking cold water and hot green tea as well. These things help your body burn extra calories images day propensity to gain weight without much of an effort.

Changes in Activity Level

Muscle mass and metabolism are not the only things affected by hormonal changes present in the bodies of women over 50. As progesterone, it is producer lower level. This may cause symptoms of tiredness and increase the amount of fat stored on your hips and arms. Many women over 50 fine that they need to increase their exercise regimens and change the love to come back postmenopausal situations that typically cause weight gain. One such problem many women encounter is increased levels of cortisol in the system. Cortisol tends to reduce the amount utilized and burned off during the exercise process. Because of this, there needs to be an emphasis put on cardiovascular expenditures match with muscle-building exercises so that the correct ratio of insulin and cortisone is maintained in the body. This will help to reset the metabolism of the body.

Some women find it more difficult to exercise simply because the aging process has affected mobility and the breakdown of muscle and bone makes it more difficult to have an effective workout. This may make it necessary for women to change their exercise regimen to include lower impact cardio exercises and may necessitate the introduction of strength-building exercises. Some women find that moderate yoga exercises help increase metabolism. 15 or 20 minutes of yoga improves blood flow and assist in adding strength to your body. Your metabolism may also increase by doing moderate-intensity workouts play a fast walk or an easy bike ride. You want to be able to boost your metabolism so that weight loss and maintenance is more easily maintained.

You have to try to counter the effects of menopause and to do this. You may need to make some simple adjustments to your activity level. One way to do this is to stand instead of sitting. Best standing takes more energy than sitting. This is an easy way to build strength increase metabolism without putting a lot of stress on joints by exercising vigorously.

We Slow Down, So Should Our Calorie intake

Because many women are slowing down physically, the calorie intake needs to be reduced to coincide with the reduction of physical activity. This is as much a mental challenge as well as a physical one. Their reliance on insulin production triggers thoughts of hunger even though they are not hungry. Insulin is released into the bloodstream to attach itself to glucose molecules that result from eating foods that convert to sugar, such as carbohydrates. The reduction of carbohydrates in your body will reduce the amount of insulin released into your body and can be a very effective way to lose weight. No matter whether you reduce your carbohydrates or not, you will generally need to reduce the number of calories that you're consuming because your body is working on an efficiently as you age and does not need as many calories. at the same time, normal aches and pains may reduce the amount of physical activity that you are experiencing each day. your food consumption must take into account any decreases in physical activity. one of the main ways that women gain weight after menopause is because they fail to reduce the number of calories consumed nor do they adjust their exercise regimen.

Reduced Flexibility and Restricted Movement

It is important to recognize that as the body ages, there will be increase experiences of muscle fatigue achy joints, and, unfortunately, injuries. There must be a special emphasis placed on remaining flexible and increasing flexibility to maintain good movement and flexible joints. The reason that flexibility is lost is that the tendons and collagen in the body tend to break down over time. This, along with the loss of muscle mass and bone loss from reducing rates of estrogen, make it important to maintain flexibility through warming up and stretching throughout the day. Before exercising, you should warm up so that you assist your body in easing into a range of exercises and waking up your muscles and so that they are not shocked by the impact of the exercise itself.

When you are exercising after menopause, it's a good idea to focus on resistance training and building muscle mass. Because there is a tendency to lose muscle, focusing on exercises to gain muscle will not increase bulk but maintain the muscle that is already there. By emphasizing strength training, your body will become fitter and more easily tolerate the new chemical makeup of your body. At the same time, if you're increasing your exercise, it may be necessary to rest your muscles for a day or two between workouts. Because of the susceptibility to injury, your tissues and joints may need more time to recover than you're used to after a strenuous workout. This may be eliminated with a good warm-up and a good cool down before and after your workout sessions. Be sure to focus on your range of motion while you're working out so that you are continuing to improve your flexibility so that you may grow old gracefully and be able to continue exercising across many more decades.

Food Sensitivity

Many adults develop sensitivity to foods as they get older. These may be foods that you haven't even you for all of your life, and several and they turn against you. These sensitivities occur because your body is changing. You may have less acid in your stomach to digest foods and last water in your system to dilute alcohol which may be formed from in a variety of foods. food sensitivity and intolerances can cause digestive issues like cramping and diarrhea. This makes it difficult to pinpoint what it's causing the distress. Many times, these elements are attributed to the other factors and may not be considered as sensitivity are allergies to food. When adults find the day become allergic to dairy products, wheat, and soy over time. These allergies may also cause heart and respiratory problems as well as sleep issues. many times, people consider the issues as typical to aging and do not associate discomfort with food allergies or sensitivities. If you find that you are consistently uncomfortable with eating certain foods, it is better to be tested for allergies. You may not feel that the allergy is life-threatening, but they can be. Living with food allergies is difficult, but you will feel better if you're able to avoid allergens in your diet.

Consumption of Processed Foods

Processed foods can adversely affect your diet and even your exercise routines. Any processed foods' powerful assault orange ball spike your blood pressure, and even in moderation, they can cause weight gain and discomfort. That may not be convenient, but pre-packaged foods are not always a good option for a diet. It's better to know what you're eating, by reading labels in preparing food from raw materials in your kitchen. This gives you control over your food intake in your diet.

When you are purchasing prepared foods for the sake of convenience, you may be eliminating some items from your diet that are necessary. Even foods that some of the nutritional value of that you're purchasing. Take, for example, bagged lettuce. This lettuce is often treated; it was a wash of bleach and water to eliminate bugs and debris from the lettuce. Well, we can all imagine that we don't want bugs in our veggies, the bleach may clear away bacteria that are helpful in our digestive system. This may cause gastrointestinal issues. By avoiding processed foods, you're forcing yourself and your body to be healthy. Eating foods that have not been processed that you can feel yourself is a good way to avoid dieting. You know what you're eating because it takes more time, I want to be more thoughtful about what year praying to your body and how it will affect you. It will take research to be sure that you are consuming all the vitamins or nutrients necessary, but this is a way to avoid vitamin supplements and diet aids. You can get all the nutrients that you need through food. Avoiding packaged and processed foods will help you to have energy and be healthier.

Latent Sensitivity Becomes Active

Sometimes when we keep the same foods over and over again, sensitivity becomes apparent. Think of it as having a limited amount of one type of food that your body can tolerate over a lifetime. Once you reach that point, you cannot eat it without breaking out into a rash are experiencing respiratory distress. This may be the result of eating a lot of a certain type of food or maybe just a little., In the end, the food must be eliminated. Many people do not consider the possibility of allergies and do not seek attention for this type of food issue. This is what happens when sensitivity becomes an allergy. Many people can eat foods throughout their lifetime; it suddenly it must be avoided.

Reduction of Muscle Mass

Muscle mass is reduced as women go through menopause. If you are exercising regularly throughout menopause and post-menopause. To limit the reduction of muscle mass, it is important to exercise. you may need to switch your exercise routines to focus on building muscle and maintaining muscle. As you grow older, the estrogen levels decrease and the loss of those are not being assisted and maintaining their mass as they were when estrogen levels were higher.

Over the age of 50, women begin to lose muscle mass at a rate of 3% per year. The loss of muscle mass is the result of several factors aside from the drop in estrogen levels. A sedentary lifestyle is a good cause of losing muscle mass. You can begin to lose muscle quickly by not using your muscles. For this reason, it is important to stay active and use as many muscles as possible and keep moving. It is also common for a poor diet to cause a loss of muscle. This happens two women over 50 because of changes in what is easily digested as you get older. Some people may find it difficult to get out and buy groceries; it may not feel like cooking and preparing food, and in the end, they eat poorly.

Other chronic illnesses may make it difficult to maintain muscle mass. There are difficulties in movement, like issues caused by arthritis, so it may be difficult to continue to maintain the muscle mass that you may have experienced earlier in life. Any health condition that makes it difficult to exercise will have an idea to have a fact on maintaining muscle mass. If you're relatively healthy, be sure to work at maintaining muscle mass because it will make you look and feel better. By incorporating strength training into your lifestyle, you'll find it easier to burn calories and maintain your way, your memory be improved, and your muscles be stronger as well as your bones. Strength exercises are a good way to avoid the development of osteoporosis.

Adults over the age of 40 tend to lose about a pound of muscle mass per year. This can easily be offset with regular exercise. It is important not to fall into the trap of thinking that you cannot do anything to change your body. Yes, he does take its toll on the body. At the same time, you can offset those changes, and you should start making those changes in your life. even if you have already begun to lose muscle mass, beginning a strength training routine allows you to build back the muscle lost and add on to it. It's not too late to offset some of the changes that may have already occurred. The way to build muscle mass is to revert to the old exercises and techniques. Get on the rowing machine in a row to build muscle mass in your arms and legs. Weightlifting and sit-ups will firm your muscles and increase the muscle mass as well. You may want to work out with lighter weights more often or increasing the number of reps. This will build your muscles slowly and not provide excess bulk to your muscles. The goal is to have muscles that support you and provide a framework for the next decades of your life. You don't have too heavy work. You just need to use your muscles until they are tired. That is how the muscle is strengthened and the mass is increased.

Increase in Protein Consumption

It is important to increase your protein consumption when you are trying to gain muscle mass and lose weight. The proteins consumed should be lean proteins that will help to build the muscles and increase the collagen within the ligaments and tendons.

There are many ways to introduce lean protein into your diet, even if there is no animal protein. The best way to do this is to combine various forms of grain and seed protein so that you are consuming the recommended daily amount of protein regularly. This may be done by mixing a grain, like oatmeal, and a seed, like flaxseed for a breakfast that is high in fiber and protein but does not include animal protein. By mixing the sources of protein, your body is better able to absorb the protein directly into the areas where it is needed.

Protein will also help with increasing and maintaining bone density. Protein can be a vital source of healthfulness as women age. Eating foods that are full of good proteins is necessary, and women who have experienced menopause should have at least four servings of protein each day. This may include soy products, which are rich in protein, and beans, and nuts. Foods high in lysine, an amino acid, are particularly necessary. The lysine assists the body in absorbing protein. Some of the foods high in lysine are avocados, leeks, peppers, mangos, beans, tofu, pumpkin seeds, macadamia nuts, and quinoa. Combine these foods with protein-rich foods like black beans, corn, oats, guava, and chickpeas. Many dairy products, like Greek yogurt and cottage cheese, are also high in protein. These products can be found made with almond or soy milk and remain consistent with a plant-based diet.

Consuming four servings of protein each day will do a lot to help maintain the ability to gain muscle and strengthen bones in women over the age of fifty. It is sometimes difficult to imagine that plants contain protein, but many do. Fortunately, many contain a sufficient amount of protein to be considered healthy and can be eaten to build muscles, especially when combined with exercise.

Weightlifting Exercises

Weightlifting is important for women over the age of 50. Lifting weights will increase your metabolism and strengthen your bones and your muscles.as you add muscle, you'll also be burning fat. Weightlifting is the most effective way to improve your health 1 basic type of exercise.

For most people, after the age of 50, you will want to increase the number of reps completed for each muscle group you're exercising. This world means that you are using lighter weights and perhaps doing different types of exercises for the same muscle group. This is where weight training with machines can come in handy. You will be able to move from machine-to-machine work on the same basic muscle groups, but you may be able to work on top of the muscle or the bottom by simply changing your grip or utilizing the machine in a slightly different manner. Make sure you give your muscles time to recover after a workout. You may need two to three days of rest for each muscle group before you work out again. Most people workout back and legs one day house in chest another or some combination. Use weights that are light enough to comfortably do up to 20 repetitions. at the end of the exercise, your muscles should be tired, but you should still be able to move them; it's not feeling any pain or strain as a result of the exercise. Conditioning workouts with a good stretch. This will give your muscles of opportunity to be there more flexible and improve overall movement and recovery time after you work out.

For people who do not belong to a gym or may not have an ability or desire to work out in a communal setting, a full home gym is not necessary to get a good workout at home. There are a variety of workouts available on the internet and various streaming services for at-home workouts. It is always possible to utilize items you have at your home to lift a weight. You can do a lot with just a few dumbbells at our home. Start with small weights and practice using the proper form to get the most out of your workout. There are many activities, like calisthenics, that can be done in your home to strengthen your core abdominal muscles, arm, and leg muscles. Walking up and down a set of stairs at a brisk pace is a good way to ward off extra weight and minimize the effects of aging. Start slowly, if you are not accustomed to exercising, and gradually increase the amount of effort you exert in doing the exercises. It is important to maintain a regular schedule and continuously exercise all the muscle groups you can. Building muscle takes time and effort. By putting forth a good effort, you will be able to feel better and healthier over time. Introduce new exercises gradually as you become comfortable with your accomplishments. Exercising will be more pleasant if it is not overly repetitive.

By adding strength and flexibility to your body, you will be pleased with the results. Improved balance and steadiness are often the results of strengthening your abdominal muscles. You will be steadier on your feet with stronger muscles in your thighs and calves. The muscles in your arms will show the most physical difference. You may not have the defined muscles of a thirty-year-old who spends hours each day in the gym, but you should be able to see the muscles start to develop over time. Overall, your general health will be improved, and that is just as important, if not more important, than improved appearance.

Chapter 2: Do You Need to Change Your Thoughts About Food and Exercise?

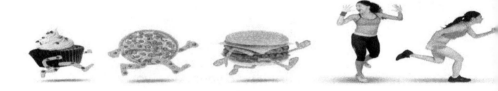

One of the difficulties in aging is that it may be necessary to change habits you had for most of your adult life. This is not easy for most people. Even if you have led a relatively healthy and fit lifestyle, aging may make it necessary to modify lifestyle choices you have always used successfully in the past. This is simply because your body is changing, and with it, you may we can make some changes. This is not an easy task for everyone. First, you have to accept that what you've always done is not working as well as it always has. Secondly, you have to want to make the changes. You may be accepting of your new padding around your hips and your stomach, so you have to make a conscious effort to change your diet exercise because of the general health ramifications of carrying extra weight. You also need to be conscious of the overall health Miss of carrying extra weight and of losing muscle mass and bone density. It is important to accept that hourly you may appear fine. You may not even feel bad as you go about your day, but you need to make an effort to have tests performed to verify that you are as healthy as you feel.

Food as Fuel, Not Fun

For many people, food represents more than nourishment. Entire industries are built upon the concept that food makes you feel good. There is an emphasis on good tasting food, and I'm consuming products that make you feel good. To have a healthy thought process running food, you need to start thinking of food as fuel, instead of a means of enjoyment. Will you look at how you relate to food, you may begin to understand why you may need to change your thoughts about food.

Many people have grown up with food as a reward for specific behaviors. This translates into access to many people as they grow into adults. Food is a way to control your happiness. If you are always offered a cookie for completing a task eating all your food and dinner, it may be natural for you to the all the cookies you want when you're brought up and be happy to do it because you want a cookie. You may even be rewarding yourself for a job well done. Even if you have broken that have it when you're raising your children, you may not have rewarded your children with food, but you may in the back of your mind reward yourself with food or a glass of wine after a hard day of work. just because you reward yourself with an adult beverage does that make the action any different in theory. Take time to think about how you feel about food and understand if you are indulging calorie consumption that does that help you in any way. Limit your option of food items that do not contribute to your healthy body. If you're going to eat a treat, it's better to have a treat with some nutritional value something filled with empty calories in the form of sugar. It's important to relegated food to a scientific organism designed to feed the body and nourish your muscles. Minimize the over-indulgences of the holidays and special occasions. If you wean yourself off of sugary treats and high carbohydrate items, you will find that your mental and physical state improves, including the ability to sleep longer and better.

Forget Comfort Food, Find a Hobby

Many people find that as they age, they are relying on food to provide excitement and relaxation in their lives. This is not a good idea. This turns food into your enemy because there is a tendency to indulgent foods that may have limited nutritional value. Thinking about food all the time rarely has a positive effect on your physical body. Channel all that energy you are spending on thinking about what you can't have into a hobby. Find something you like to do that keeps you busy and can be incorporated into other activities as well. If you develop a hobby like needlepoint, you will be able to keep your hands moving and concentrate on something other than eating. A hobby may even be combined with travel.so you have a reason to visit places that don't necessarily revolve around eating. Especially if you have a sedentary lifestyle, it is important to limit the number of calories consumed. That is a lot easier if you have something to occupy your thoughts. The idea is to find comfort in something besides food. Do something that makes you feel good and doesn't involve food.

For many people will be necessary to modify their diet as they age. This may have the unwanted effect of considering limits to your diet as deprivation. Rather than think of your new diet requirements as rules and restrictions, it is better to think your food as fuel to help your body efficiently work for you throughout the day. Try to avoid thinking about food as a stress reliever. Food consumed to release stress is generally high in sugar and fat. This releases endorphins into the system that makes us feel good temporarily. Mentally, we may feel good, but usually but there is a mental and physical swim after consumption. Consuming the fat and sugar spikes the blood sugar and cortisol levels in the blood but they are quickly dissipated, which causes a dramatic drop in blood sugar levels.

Eating foods to change your mood is a learned behavior. Modify your thoughts and actions so that you resort to other, less unhealthy, ways to deal with stress and unhappiness. For some people, this is easier to do. For others, it is very difficult. No matter whether it's easy or difficult, you must try to channel inappropriate relationships with food until appropriate relationships with.

When Did This Whole Comfort Food Philosophy Come About?

You probably started thinking about food as a comfortable feeling in your childhood. on special occasions may have had the opportunity to pick your favorite meal and eat your favorite cake. The celebration foods hold an array of meanings for people. Celebration foods historical and traditional for people of all cultures. To recreate good feelings of family gatherings, many people relate the food. It's off to the Good feeling instead of the people in comradery. This has led to "comfort food" as a phenomenon. Eating these foods may cause allow for temporary relief of stress. But the fact is, the feeling is only temporary. To relieve stress, it is better to find a productive activity that assists you in dealing with stress and coping with stressful situations. It may be that your new hobby is exercise. By combining the correct exercise to your lifestyle and body type, this could be the best way to combat health issues as your body adjust to being over 50.

Limit Alcohol Consumption

There are a few reasons to limit alcohol consumption as you age. Primarily the reasons have to do with health concerns. Women tend to process alcohol more slowly than when men consume alcohol. What are the reasons is because alcohol dissolves in water, and women have less water in their bodies than men do? Coupled with the decrease in bone density, consuming alcohol may simply not be as safe for women. Intoxication may quickly demonstrate its whimsy to some women because of the state of the body after menopause.

Falls and broken bones are more common in women over the age of 50.

Consuming alcohol regularly can also increase diseases such as liver disease, depression, is some types of cancer. This is especially true for heavy drinkers. Moreover, alcohol consumption may turn until carbohydrates and the fact your insulin production in your body. This is especially true for beer drinkers and those who drink mixed drinks with sweetened mixes and juices. there's a growing number of women who are having problems with alcohol consumption. consuming alcohol lowers your inhibitions and reduces your ability to make sound judgments. So, even if it's a simple food choice, one should have the clarity of mind to make good food choices instead of compounding bad choices on top of that choice. of course, moderate consumption of wine and other alcoholic beverages may have beneficial effects on your health. It is important to limit your consumption to those that are beneficial. It's not a bad thing to drink one glass of wine per day, and avoid binge drinking and excess consumption of alcohol. Alcohol does that metabolize while in your system, and excessive amounts of alcohol will hurt your body over time.

In a nutshell, consuming alcohol to the point of intoxication can we two a decrease in stability and physical acumen. Being tipsy can lead to falls both inside the home and outside the home. This can lead to bones breaking do the tenancy for bones in women over 50 to be more brittle and less dense than they were previously in a woman's life. Additionally, consuming high amounts of alcohol can lead to medical issues such as liver disease and some types of cancer. As far as that goes, one or two glasses of wine did you just stay might medically advantageous. But overall, the consumption of alcohol can cause more problems than it solves.

Many people believe that consuming alcohol will increase their ability to sleep. This is not true. Alcohol consumption while affects the quality of sleep that you have. You may pass out and consider this as sleeping, but you will not feel refreshed in the morning as your body will suffer from dehydration and fitful sleep cycles. Many types of alcohol consumed, especially wind, contains a lot of sugar that will keep you awake at night.

Chemical Preservatives Are for Chumps

As you get older, it's important to monitor what you are introducing into your body. After the age of 50, you may want to switch to organic foods and have a good idea of what is included in the food that you're consuming. Chemical preservatives are not useful for your diet.

One reason to eliminate chemical preservatives for your diet is that most preservatives are derivative from some form of salt or sodium. The excess sodium that you'll find in these preservatives are unhealthy and cause weight gain for water retention and bloating. Especially true for lunch meats and deli meats. Many of these means that you may find either pre-packaged or at the deli of your local store are probably served using sodium and may have been injected with fats which flavor to the meat products. Let's face it, pre-packaged foods are convenient and easy to prepare. We all need some of these items in our pantries in freezers to be able to big healthy meals with busy schedules. Being unable to eliminate processed foods from her diet is an issue for many people today. The best thing to do is to read the ingredients on the items and be sure to purchase foods that are organically grown and naturally preserved. For instance, frozen vegetables should be simply that vegetables. There is no need to add additional chemicals are salt to these vegetables. It is also preferable to purchase organic products. this is important so that you're not consuming chemicals through fertilization and drawing techniques that matrix Hammond in your plant-based diet.

Exercise Is Not Just for Health Nuts

It is simply not possible to avoid the need for exercise as we age. Changes in the body make it necessary to modify previous exercise patterns and institute in an exercise regime if you are not already involved in one. The loss of muscle mass in women over 50 is a real issue. This occurs because the estrogen levels AR decrease, and the proteins are not as easily absorbed into the muscle. The protein helps to build muscle and as estrogen levels decrease, it is harder for women to maintain muscle mass. Because mobility often decreases after the age of 50, women are not as likely to take on new exercises due to pain, decreased flexibility, and lack of protein consumption.

Start Early, Before it Gets Worse

It's never too early to start exercising. at the same time, it's not too late either. It's a good idea to see if its position before beginning an exercise program to be sure what exercise do you need to emphasize and how often your doctor feels will be able to exercise. By starting to exercise early, you will be able to maintain flexibility have a good

47

chance to maintain muscle mass as well. Bone density and joint health may also be positively affected by a well-planned exercise schedule. By starting to exercise early, you'll be in the habit of exercise and may easily be able to make transitions to postmenopausal exercises necessary to maintain adequate muscle and bone health.

Exercise for Mental Health and Physical

Exercise is always a good mental health plan because it helps relieve stress and activate endorphins, which provide feelings of happiness after your workout. Using the time while you work out as an opportunity to mentally recharge is a good way to multi-task. Exercise may be a way to release chemical happiness into your bloodstream. Taking the time to exercise for health will also promote a healthy mental attitude as well.

It is harder for women over 50 to use protein to build muscle mass. the ability to build muscle mass decreases even further by the time a woman reaches the age of 65. Therefore, it is important to be in the habit of exercising and working on producing muscle in your workouts. This is often done through anaerobic exercises like yoga and other forms of strength training. The frequency of these workouts may vary, but the exercise important for overall health improvement.

Chapter 3: Reset Your Diet to Plant-Based

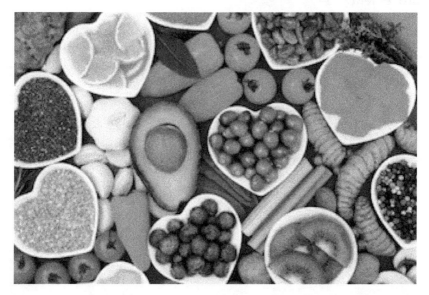

If you have not previously considered a plant-based diet, there are several reasons why this can be an ideal time of life to make the switch, especially if you have not yet gone through menopause. The change to a plant-based diet has specific benefits for women over 50. At a time when many women experience increases in anxiety due to changes in life circumstances and health, many of the benefits of a plant-based diet will help to alleviate the symptoms of menopause and the general aging process.

Reduce Carbohydrates

Many women over the age of 50 find that they are gaining weight and lacking energy. This may partly be due to the consumption of carbohydrates at the wrong time of day and from the wrong foods. It is important to eliminate the most detrimental carbohydrates, like those derived from dairy and sugar, to be able to achieve a comfortable and healthy weight without added stress on organs like the liver.

Carbohydrates are the primary source of energy in the average diet. When you eat carbohydrates, they are converted into energy with the excess being stored in your liver. Therefore, carbohydrates are needed to provide energy. When you are physically active, your body uses the energy from carbohydrates quickly and efficiently. Problems occur when the energy is not used, and the stored energy is converted to fat. Adults over the age of 50 need to eat about 130 grams of carbohydrates daily. When you eat more carbs than the recommended daily amount, you have to work off the extra carbs. With only 130 carbohydrates, it is necessary to be sure to eat the most useful carbs and avoid carbs that harm your body.

Carbs Add Weight

Carbohydrates can be a source of weight gain, especially when they contain excessive amounts of fat and calories. Some of the things we consume regularly can be high in carbohydrates and fat, which add to unwanted weight gain.

Coffee has many healthful properties and can be a source of antioxidants and has properties to combat liver disease, type-2 diabetes, and certain types of cancer. That is what coffee can do for you...until you turn it into a dessert with sugar, fatty cream, and sticky syrups. Black coffee has virtually no calories and no carbohydrates. Stick to the basics and coffee has qualities that can increase metabolism without impinging upon your healthy diet plan.

Another carb-heavy form of drink that starts healthy is the current trend of smoothies. Though fruit is good for you in moderation, the concentration of high-sugar fruits in some smoothies eliminates the healthful properties of the smoothie. It is beneficial if there are at least twice as many vegetable ounces in your smoothies as fruit. Use a vegetable juice or ice to provide the liquid aspect of the smoothie instead of fruit juice or a dairy base.

White bread, bagels, and crackers tend to be empty calories. They provide little nutritional value. They are filling while eating them, but they generate energy that burns quickly and do not provide sustained energy that we need to last throughout the day. Whole grains are best in a situation where you need to eat a bread option. The whole grains last longer as an energy source. Let go of the white bread, which can be upwards of half your carbohydrates allowed for the day. Many of the over-processed white bread products contain high fructose corn syrup and add to the calories and carbohydrates. Stick with whole-grain bread that is filling and has good nutritional values.

White rice is broken down into just starch. Like white bread, the process of making rice white eliminates the vitamins and fiber contained in the grain. The most healthful aspects of rice are on the husks that are removed during processing. It's better to eat brown rice, which has decent nutritional value.

Another vegetable that has lost its healthy properties is the potato in the form of fries. The nutritional goodness of the potato is mainly in the skin. When the potato is peeled and fried, much of the fiber is lost, and the nutritional value is diminished. A better option is to eat sweet potato fries that have less than half the calories and less than

60% of the carbohydrates. The sweet potato is a better alternative to the white potato, even when you're making fries.

Other carbohydrates are common in today's diet. Snack foods like chips and pretzels have little nutritional value and lots of calories and carbohydrates. It is better to snack on kale chips and dried sugar snap peas. Another alternative is dried seaweed. These items provide a satisfying crunch with vitamins and fiber.

As we age, the carbohydrates we consume need to be more efficient and richer in fiber and nutrients. The body is not as forgiving, and we are often less able to provide our bodies with vigorous exercise that may assist in burning off excess carbohydrates. By concentrating on eating better carbs while keeping the 130-carbohydrate maximum recommended, you will take the first step in eliminating excess weight and minimize the likelihood of weight gain resulting from foods high in sugar, dairy, and fat.

Eliminate Animal Fats

If you are wondering why it is preferable to reduce the amount of animal fat consumed, it is basically because animal fats are not healthy, and in any diet, should be consumed in moderation. While all fats should be monitored, the reduction of animal fat from your diet may be a good way to improve your health and lower your bad cholesterol levels. We all need to have a certain level of fat in our diets. Monounsaturated fats are often considered to be "good fats." They are found in seeds, nuts, and vegetable oils. They are high in HDL cholesterol which is good for the heart, and low in LDL cholesterol, which causes thickening of arteries and has been linked to high rates of heart disease and stroke. The fats with good cholesterol are those found in plants are monounsaturated fats and can be found in avocados, macadamia nuts, olives, olive oil, peanuts, peanut oil, canola oil, and pecans. Good fats are also polyunsaturated fats, which can be found in tofu, sunflower seeds, pumpkin seeds, flaxseed, and sesame seeds. These are all plant-based fats that are high in good cholesterol. They should be a fixture in your daily diet. The chart below indicates the recommended amount of fat grams that should be included. The number of saturated fats should not exceed the recommended amount, even if it less than the total fat grams.

Saturated fats are those found in red meat, chicken skin, lard, whole-fat dairy, and ice cream. These fats raise LDL levels and can be a protagonist in unhealthy heart health. By following a plant-based diet, these fats will be eliminated from your diet. There are a few plant-based saturated fats, like palm oil and coconut oil. These should be used in moderation.

It will also be a good idea to eliminate trans fats from your diet as they have the same or similar effects as saturated fats on the body. They are usually found in processed foods as they are used stabilizers and extend the shelf-life of foods. Trans fats are often found in packaged snacks and pastries. They are also common in microwave popcorn and stick margarine. Also, partially hydrogenated and hydrogenated oil is usually a trans-fat no matter what the packaging says.

Limit the consumption of saturated and trans fats so that there are fewer amounts of LDL cholesterol generated. This allows the fats consumed that produce HDL to do a good job of limiting the production of LDL while allowing the good fat to be stored in the muscle as energy.

Calories each Day	Fat in Grams per day	Sat. Fat in Grams per day

1,200 kilocalories	40g	13g
1,600 kilocalories	53g	18g
2,000 kilocalories	67g	22g

Nutritional labels differentiate between saturated fats and total fats. It is important that when limited saturated fats and trans-fats, there is not an exchange for another food that should not be included in your diet if your goal is to improve overall health. If we keep in mind that eliminating pork breakfast sausage is a good idea, but that breakfast item should not be replaced with another unhealthful food choice. For example, if you are eliminating bacon and sausage from your diet and you want to replace it with a plant-based item and decide on toast made with white bread, this is not an exchange that will result in the most healthful meal, even though it doesn't include meat or dairy. The better replacement would be a whole oat porridge mixed with flaxseed or chia seeds. This will produce fiber and nutrients while providing energy to get started with your day. Removing butter, meat, and milk products will be necessary for adopting a plant-based diet. By eliminating dairy from your diet, you are essentially eliminating a form of saturated fat. For dairy products, you may want to replace milk and yogurt with almond, soy, or oat milk products.

almond products are very popular but do not act like dairy products. Almond milk does not have as much calcium or fast as cow's milk, so it is considered a popular alternative to house milk. Soy products and soy milk have more calcium than almond milk and are still lower in calories than cow's milk. Many soy products have added nutrients so that the nutritional value of the product is similar to that of cow's milk. This makes soya a good replacement if there is an allergy to soy products. Luckily, soy products are available in milk and yogurt, and often can be a good substitute for milk and yogurt products. There are plant-based products that can be substituted for cream cheese, sour cream, and butter. Many of these products are derived from almond or soy. There are also products based on cashew, pea, hemp, and oats.

Avoid Hormones and Antibiotics

One of the primary reasons to convert to a plant-based diet will be to eat clean. By eating clean, you will restrict certain foods from your diet. These foods are those containing animal hormones antibiotics and other chemical additives that are often used to assist in speeding the growth of the food and prolonging the shelf life of the food. When you are transitioning to a diet that is the healthiest possible, you'll want to avoid antibiotics and hormones.

Some of the guest mental effects of the seas hormones which are fed to animals in the meat industry have to do with inhibiting the growth of good bacteria in the digestive system human to consume these animal products. The use of these hormones can be perfectly legal and promote the health and growth of the animals that will be consumed by humans. At the same time, they do affect the humans consuming the products, which generally manifest themselves in gastro internal distress.

Eliminating animal products from your diet is a way to eliminate the stress of figuring out whether animal hormones will affect your body. Realistically, if the hormones are affecting anal meat, it is also going to affect the milk and the products resulting from the milk like butter, cream, and cheese. For this reason, there is good reason to avoid eating all animal products.

The use of chemicals in animals has been linked to increases in the rate of some breast cancers, prostate, and other cancers. This is linked to a chemical Insulin-like Growth Factor, or IGF, which mimics growth hormones in cows and may be used as a replacement for growth hormones. The modern process of producing dairy products has created an industry that is allowed to create an artificially "safe" speeding of producing food which allows farm companies to get food to market faster than ever. The food is bigger and may be promoted as being more nutritious. The fact is, the chemicals added to foods through the source animals are not always safe and it may take years to determine the effects of additives and the effects on humans. This has been the impetus of the growth in sales of organic products.

Organic products should be sought when your focus is a plant-based diet. fertilizer used to promote plant growth may also include some antibiotics and hormone type chemicals to promote the bigger, faster crop rotation proliferation. So, when you're looking to adopt a clean diet, try to focus on eating foods that have minimal additives or if there are attitude tips to the food that they are natural and organic. There is a long history of farming and agriculture, and over time there have been developments in organic gardening that promote healthy non-toxic additives to your food supply that do not make your food likely to be unhealthful for you. Part of the problem with the food like the recent rash of E Coli issues makes it important to purchase produce that is grown without infected animal products used as fertilizer. So, when you're looking at purchasing organic products, be sure that it was processed organically from the inception through the process to it being on your table. The E Coli outbreaks on lettuce products were the result of the fertilizer coming from infected animal manure. Because produce is often eaten raw, there isn't a chance to use heat to destroy some of the bacteria microorganisms that cause issues, so especially on your raw vegetables, you need to be sure that the process of its growth has been organic and that there is less chance for contamination.

Best Plants to Consume

Switching to a plant-based diet can be a confusing proposition if meat and dairy have always been a part of your diet. You have spent 50 years of omnivorous eating, and a switch to eating only plants will entail learning more about fruit, vegetables, and grains than you have ever thought of achieving. Because you will need to know how to provide your body with nutrition-packed plants that must be satisfying and filling if you are going to adapt the diet to your forever lifestyle.

Women, over the age of 50, may want to modify the intake of certain foods to adjust to the changing requirements of their aging bodies. Here is a list of the recommended daily intake of food items and the plant-based foods that can be used to meet the required amount to eat daily:

Nutrient/Vitamin	Recommended Daily	How it nourishes	Foods to Eat
Protein	46 grams	It helps to strengthen muscle and offset the loss of muscle mass.	Beans, peas, seeds, and tofu.
Iron	8 mg	Carries oxygen in the blood so that organs get enough oxygen. Iron is necessary to stave off anemia, fatigue, and decreased immunity.	Leafy greens, legumes like beans and lentils, iron-enriched bread, dried fruit, nuts, seeds.

Vitamin D	600 international units (15mcg)	Promotes the absorption of calcium into the body.	Enriched plant-based milk.
Calcium	1,200 mg per day	Strengthens bone density to offset the loss from the decrease in estrogen.	Leafy greens, green vegetables, enriched plant-based milk, and tofu
Carbohydrate	130 grams	Provide energy to get through the day. The energy is stored in muscles in the form of glucose to be used throughout the day.	Whole grains, fruits, and beans and lentils. On a normal diet, carbohydrates should be around 40% of the daily calorie intake.

Green Leafy Vegetables

The first thing that you will need to incorporate into your diet is green leafy vegetables. These are important as a source of calcium. Since dairy will be eliminated from your diet, it will be important to draw a source of calcium to guard against bone loss, which is common for women over the age of 50. There is such an abundance of dark green leafy vegetables available to most people. It is the perfect opportunity to try out different vegetables and be able to switch between the various vegetables and experience a variety of meal options.

There is a marked difference between the various types of green leafy vegetables. It is important to consume these vegetables to attain variance nutrients, but be careful when eating a vegetable for its calcium source because some green leafy vegetables block calcium from being absorbed into the system. High oxalate vegetables do not allow the absorption of calcium into the system. These are vegetables like spinach, endive, beet tops, and Swiss chard contain vitamins in their own right, but should not be used as a source of calcium. Low oxalate vegetables like collard greens, kale, broccoli, romaine lettuce, turnip greens, and Brussel sprouts are a good source of calcium, good enough to replace dairy products in your diet. The calcium from low oxalate leafy green vegetables is more easily absorbed into the system than calcium from milk and dairy.

Aside from calcium, green leafy vegetables are a good addition to any diet. Packed with nitrates, they are known to greatly reduce cardiovascular disease, heart disease, and helpful in avoiding type 2 diabetes. The potassium in these green vegetables may help overall health, working as an anti-inflammatory. The vitamin K in these leafy vegetables is beneficial in preventing blood clots and assist in strengthening bones. This is especially useful for women over 50 to offset the bone loss associated with the lack of estrogen after menopause.

One nutrient that women do not need as much after menopause is iron. Because menstruation has ended, there is not an associated loss of iron. Accordingly, post-menopausal women need less iron than women of childbearing years. This is best accomplished on a plant-based diet by eating green leafy vegetables in combination with beans and other iron-rich foods. The iron is most easily absorbed in the system when it is combined with vitamin C. So, it is best to accompany your iron-rich vegetable with a vitamin C rich item. Magnesium is also a mineral found in green leafy vegetables. The magnesium helps maintain strong muscles, regulate blood sugar and the nervous system, and even assisting in bone development.

Green leafy vegetables are the backbone of a plant-based diet because they are instrumental in providing vitamins, minerals, and nutrients that provide healthy bodies and nutrition. Some of the vegetables are best raw. Others provide nutrition that is more easily absorbed into your body when cooked. It is best to have a variety of cooked and raw vegetables in several meals throughout your week. The fiber in the vegetables will also help to clean your arteries and flush your gastrointestinal system. Green leafy vegetables are a superfood that will provide a vast amount of nutrition for a healthy diet which will, in the end, provide energy, strong muscles, and strong bones.

Hard Crunch Vs. Liquid Nutrition

When you start to change to a plant-based diet, feeling satisfied will be the best way to successfully transition from the diet of an omnivore. There is a great deal of satisfaction in eating, and the pleasure we receive from food varies from person to person and meal to meal. Be sure to get the most out of your calories. Make sure what you eat is both filling, as well as nutrient-dense.

Studies show that your brain considers crunchy foods more satisfying than soft foods. The prevailing thought is that crunchy foods take more time to eat. Because of all of the chewing and time spent eating, your brain has time to recognize being full, and the food is more satisfying. Our brain considers the first few bites of food as the best tasting. The pleasure of eating decreases with each subsequent bite of food. By the time you are finished eating a full serving of food, the brain recognizes satisfaction with the serving of food. Why are we talking about chewing food? Well, because it may be tempting to load a blender or juicer with a variety of fruits and vegetables and pulverize your breakfast. A blended drink is a good way to get a lot of nutrients, vitamins, and minerals into your diet in a possibly delicious concoction.

The problem with smoothies and juices are similar. Smoothies, even if they do not include dairy, may include plant-based sweeteners to improve the taste. This adds calories and may not be as satisfying as eating the foods included in the smoothie. Juices may eliminate a lot of the natural fiber that is included in fruits and vegetables. So, even if you are not adding sugar or sweetener, some of the nutrients are eliminated from the foods during the juicing process. It is better to eat the food as part of your meal rather than drinking your meal.

Chewing your food takes more time, and by chewing and eating slowly, the brain can sense the feeling of fullness. On the other hand, smoothies made in blenders break down the cell walls of fruits and vegetables. This makes digestion easier because the food is already partially broken down. The act of chewing and mastication is a required part of the digestive process. The fine chop of the fruits and veggies in the blender cannot be recreated by chewing. For chewing food to be the same, it would necessitate chewing food until it is liquid. Unfortunately, the body may not recognize fullness right away, because smoothies tend to be consumed quickly, not allowing the brain to trigger the sensors controlling fullness and satisfaction.

Because smoothies can include a lot of vegetables and fruits that are broken down, the nutrients are easily absorbed into your bloodstream. You can include a variety of nutritious foods in your smoothie, including seeds, fruits, and vegetables. If you take the time to sip the drink, you give your brain time to register that you are eating and filling up your stomach. Do not add fruit juice and water to your smoothie. Watery additives do not remain in the body for as long as solid foods. The foods used in your smoothie should include the fibrous, edible parts of the foods. This will give good fiber, which will remain longer in your stomach and give your body time to soak up the nutrients before being evacuated from the body.

What About Sugar?

You may consider that sugar, as long as you stay below your daily calorie requirements, is fair game. As long as the sugar is derived from plants, you will be staying with the recommended guidelines, and it will be healthy. Unfortunately, other factors of sugar may disrupt this theory.

Processed sugar has an aging effect on the body. It can cause type-2 diabetes, diminish the function of the brain, and damage the function of the heart. It is important to limit the consumption of refined sugars. This is another reason to eliminate processed foods from your diet. If you prepare your food with raw materials, you will be able to control the amount of sugar consumed and limit sugar intake to fresh fruits.

Many juices, especially those from concentrate, are loaded with sugar. The amount of sugar serves to regulate the flavor and provide a consistent flavor profile. Most of the "flavor" of these juices is sugar. When you are preparing beverages for yourself, make sure they are unsweetened. Use fresh when possible. I fresh fruit is not possible, try frozen.

If you are making a smoothie, many times, a recipe will call for apple juice. If you use apple juice in making smoothies, consider using an apple instead. This will change the texture of the smoothie, especially if you leave the skin on, but using a fresh apple and frozen fruit should provide enough liquid to make the smoothie thin enough to drink. Add water, to thin it out instead of juice. Consider an unsweetened, flavored seltzer to add a new dimension, sparkle, to your smoothie.

Do not overuse artificial sweeteners. Because they do not have calories, the body does not register the need to provide energy. It may stall your metabolism as a result. Even artificial sweeteners derived from sugar and not good for your body. They are processed foods that the body may consider a toxin. The processing of the artificial sweetener sometimes causes the body to battle the chemical elements of the sweetener ad may, therefore, increase inflammation within the body. Inflammation attacks joints in the body, increasing the risk for arthritis, but also has a negative impact that may lead to heart disease, attack brain function, and may have a link to some forms of cancer.

The best way to avoid hidden sugar is to eliminate processed foods from your diet. If you will continue to eat processed foods, be sure to learn all the different forms of sugar takes when you are studying food labels. There are many names for sugar. Hopefully, if you think it's too difficult to eliminate processed foods, you will find foods with easily defined ingredients that clearly state what is included in the products you are purchasing.

How Will I Replace Meat?

One of the benefits of switching to a plant-based diet is the natural reduction of saturated fats that will occur when you eliminate dairy and meat from your daily diet. This will generally improve overall cardiovascular health, and may even ward off diseases of the brain like Alzheimer's. When you eliminate meat from your diet, the protein that is found in meat products must be replaced. This leads to questions of how to receive substantial amounts of protein, especially when protein is needed to sustain muscle mass. It is recommended that women over 50 increase their protein intake to maintain and increase muscle mass. Protein also assists in helping wounds to heal and can increase communities in the body. As women get older, they do need to increase their protein levels. Protein is important for many parts of the body, including skin and nails, as well as bones and muscles. Fortunately, there are alternatives to animal products for protein, iron, and other vitamins and minerals commonly found in meat.

Soy Products

A popular alternative to animal products is soy. Soy can be used in many of the same ways and applications as meat, and that's what makes it a common go-to for meat replacement in recipes and daily. it is recommended that postmenopausal women consume at least for portions of protein-dense foods each day. This includes soy products. Soy products include soy as a raw plant and also process in the form of tofu and soy milk. Soy house to produce structures in your system that mimic estrogen, which helps to lower the risk of breast cancer after menopause. Because soy is available in many different forms, it's easy to add it to your diet in many different meals and snacks.

Protein from soy products contains all the amino acids needed by your body to build muscle. It can be a total replacement for animal protein in your diet. Adding, so it's your diet can help you improve your health and may assist in weight loss. Products like firm tofu tend to have minimal taste and take all the flavors added to it. This makes it an easy and versatile addition to many recipes. Edamame is the seed from the young soy pod and is often added to Asian cuisine. It is also roasted and flavored for snacking, similar to roasted corn products. Soy products are readily available in grocery stores which make it an easy transition from meat products.

It is recommended that soy products be limited to one to three servings daily. This is an adequate rate that will not affect the absorption of nutrients like calcium, iron, and zinc. It is best to consume less processed soy products like edamame, soy milk, and fermented soy products like miso, tempeh, and soy sauce. Processed soy products like meat-substitutes manufactured to mimic meat products for vegetarians and vegans. If you're eating these products, try to organic products without GMOs. This will make it less likely that controversial pesticides haven't been used in the growth of the soybeans. Even though so I products are plant-based, they can still be subject to the modern farming techniques that have caused illness and health concerns in the past.

Legumes and Beans

Legumes and lentils provide more than adequate vitamins and minerals, including protein, to feel your body. These vitamin-packed morsels are a wonderful way to nourish your body and provide variety to your menus and meal planning. Since there is such a vast array of beans, peas, and lentils, oh, it is easy to find ways to supplement your diet with these protein replacements. As with most things, they vary in what they bring to the table.

If you're looking for protein, chickpeas, or garbanzo beans, are the best source of protein that you will find outside of soybeans. Because of the traditional and old-world nature of garbanzo beans, these are included in the diets of individuals since ancient times. One of the more popular ratifications of the garbanzo beans is hummus, which is simply ground garbanzo beans, oil, and seasonings. Chickpeas are also known to assist in lowering blood sugar levels in individuals who consume them regularly. They are also full of fiber, which may assist in improving cholesterol levels and eating in the elimination functions of your intestines.

Chickpeas may also be ground into a flour and use instead of wheat flour as a gluten-free alternative in making bread and pasta. As long as the chickpea is organic and not subject to GMOs, it can be a healthy way to and proteins and minerals into your diet

Lentils are also a good source of plant-based protein. They can be easily added to sauces and also May reduce the risk of type 2 diabetes by reducing blood sugar levels. Reduce LDL cholesterol and increase good cholesterol in promoting an overall healthy diet.

Beans, peas, and lentils can be added into your diet and reduce the need for supplements when switching to a plant-based diet. The foods are eaten and absorbed naturally into your system without additional additives. The high-fiber aspects of legumes and lentils provide more incentive to consume the foods naturally. These foods high in fiber May assist in clearing your arteries as well as efficiently processing in your gastrointestinal system.

Replacing meat with beans provides a healthy and filling alternative to animal proteins. Unfortunately, many people experience digestive distress upon eating these items. To offset this, the feelings of bloating, constipation, diarrhea, and gas, you can add foods to your diet that contain natural enzymes to break down the foods and alleviate the associated problems of eating beans and peas. Some of the best foods to eat are various fruits. Pineapple is a good place to start to break down enzymes that help you in digesting some of the foods which may cause your stomach distress. The pineapple may also assist your body in the absorption of proteins. Papaya also has enzymes that help digestion. papaya is good to relieve constipation and bloating. That should not be cooked to receive the full benefit of the digestive enzymes. Be sure the papaya is ripe to receive the full effect.

One of the more popular methods of producing enzymes to help your body break down food in your intestinal tract is bananas. Bananas how to break down the starches in your system to a smaller size. They also add dietary fiber to help evacuate food from your system. Ripe bananas contain more the enzyme than green bananas, so used the sweetness of nature to help you with gloating.

If you're looking for a fruit to assist you that is low in sugar, avocados are the answer. Enzymes in avocado feed upon fat molecules. Though these may not help you with your gut health, it may help you to absorb fat, which can be stored as energy and help you with your overall activity levels.

In recent years, pickled foods have become popular in assisting with Digestive health through the production of probiotics. This may take the form of kimchi, sauerkraut, can kombucha. These fermented products have probiotic features which how to produce bacteria, which aids in digestion. The fermented products may also reduce appetite, total cholesterol, and also lower the risk of heart disease. The natural probiotic effect will assist in digestive function and may aid in introducing the feelings of bloating and constipation.

Ginger has long been known to help with stomach upset, and nausea. Recent studies have found that ginger assists in producing digestive enzymes so that food is processed efficiently in your system. Adding ginger to your food as a spice May produce helpful benefits in digestion as well as reducing feelings of nausea.

It is possible to add beans, peas, and lentils to your diet without having to take supplements to reduce some of the after-effects of consuming such products. There are foods which offset the uncomfortable feelings you may experience with eating beans.

Fortunately, as you reduce animal proteins in your system, reduce inflammation throughout your system assists in lessening the adverse effects of foods that may have previously produce gastrointestinal discomfort.

The Colors of My Plate

Adding a variety of colors to your plate will be instrumental in having a healthy plant-based diet. Because the color of your food demonstrates the variety of vitamins and minerals contained within it, it is important to make sure you are consuming foods with the largest array of nutritional values as possible. Since your food is all plant-based, you may think that all your food will be green. This is not true. You can add colorful vegetables to your plate, and in this way, you'll be adding vitamins and minerals to help your body flourish. Most grains tend towards the brown and beige color, which you will want to limit to approximately 25% of the daily intake of food. These grains should be whole grains when possible. Whole grains assist in digestion, reducing cholesterol, and help to ward off type 2 diabetes. Make sure to consume plenty of water while you are eating these whole grains. The water will help you with the digestion of your foods.

Some of the best ways to get more color on your plate are to think about different ways to incorporate them into your diet. The color of the food usually represents the various nutrients inside of the foods. The more colors you get on your plate, the more nutrients you will tend to eat.

Consider replacing white potatoes with sweet potatoes. They have high levels of vitamin a wish is useful and good bone health and healthy skin. This is from the beta carotene inside of the vegetables. Carrots and sweet potatoes are good suppliers of beta-carotene.

If you're looking for antioxidants and other foods promoting heart health, try adding bread foods into your diet. Some obvious red foods are cherries and watermelon but think about using other red foods like red peppers and beets. Tomatoes also fall into this category. There are snack items made from beets and sweet potatoes, and it may be easiest to supplement your diet with red foods by consuming beet chips. Cherries and watermelon have a lot of sugar in them. I may not be as useful for everyone. You can use red peppers in place of green peppers on foods and they don't have a vastly different flavor.

Blue foods like blueberries are anti-inflammatories. This can be consumed to reduce diseases of the digestive system. There are also a variety of vegetables of various colors like cauliflower, broccoli, and carrots. These new varieties tend to bring the values attributed to their color to your plate.

The new food pyramid suggests fruits and vegetables be 50% of your food consumption. Even for traditional diets, animal proteins are only recommended to be 25% of your food intake in a day. This gives you a wonderful opportunity to increase the color of your plate with produce that is readily available in most markets. Use fruits as dessert. The add to your vitamin and nutrient counts, increase your fiber intake, and do not contain the refined sugars present in baked items. Be sure to purchase organic products if possible, especially if you will be eating the skin of the fruit. Wash the fruit carefully whether it is organically grown or not. Careful selection of your fruits and vegetables well hopefully help you to select products that are flavorful and free of pesticides and bacteria.

Should You Take Supplements?

Because you'll be switching from a carnivorous processed food diet, you may find that you need to take supplements for some of the items that previously you were eating regularly. This is true because of many foods on the grocery shelves that are enriched with certain vitamins and nutrients. If you eliminate these items from your diet, you may find that certain elements are lacking. This is a reflection on the diet of the Western world in general. We tend to take for granted certain aspects of our food supply. When we switch to whole foods and minimize process foods, it may be necessary to supplement your diet with certain vitamins that you may not be receiving from the food you eat.

They're generally two vitamins that tend to be lacking in the diet of people following plant-based diets. These are vitamin B12 and vitamin d. You may be able to increase the amount included in your diet by drinking a fortified plant-based milk product. These vitamins are often added to plant-based yogurts, sour cream, and cream cheese products as well. These are items also added to conventional food products. They are because they are healthy foods for humans.

Vitamin B12 is simply not produced by plants. They're produced by fish, eggs, and meat. Deficiencies in vitamin B12 can produce atrophy of brain tissue, bone loss, and heart issues. For this reason, it is important to either supplement with a water-soluble vitamin, or make sure your processed foods contain additional vitamin B12 in the serving size.

Vitamin D is also a vitamin that is more and more, not consumed by adults. One of the best ways to add vitamin D to your body is to simply get out into the sun. Of course, most people eschew the sun to avoid the possibilities of melanoma and skin cancers. This is a problem because vitamin D serves a purpose in our bodies, and the sun is an effective source. The immune system is greatly boosted by vitamin D. There also needs to be sufficient amounts of vitamin D in your system to absorb calcium while. Since women are susceptible to bone loss after the age of 50, calcium needs to be present and absorbed to fortify our bones as efficiently as possible. Again, vitamin D is often used as a supplement in dairy products. Fortunately, non-dairy milk products have also taken to adding vitamin d to their milk, cream, yogurt, and cream cheese. if you are not consuming enough vitamin d, a supplement may be necessary for vitamin D3 to make sure that you are consuming appropriate amounts of vitamin D.

Overall, be sure to notify your physician of your dietary change so that the levels of key vitamins and nutrients are monitored. Generally, if you have a well-rounded diet, it will be easier to consume the vast array of vitamins, minerals, and nutrients necessary to maintain a healthy body.

Fried Green Tomatoes are Plant-Based—Should They Be Avoided?

We've gone over several foods that are excellent on a plant-based diet, what are some of the foods that should be avoided? It's important to understand that the foods on this list are likely to upset your system and counteract the work here doing by successfully adhering to a plant-based diet. Everything on this list of things to avoid can be considered plant-based. The issue is that these items are unhealthful and provide means of sabotage as you seek a healthy diet.

The first things that should be eliminated from your plant-based diet are processed foods. There are too many additives and chemicals hidden within the process of making the food to ignore. Though it is often convenient to consume such products, and they are often full of salt and preservatives. They may also contain sugar. The problem with the salt in the sugar included in the processed food is that they are often labeled by their chemical makeup rather than and easily defined label like salt and sugar. This includes eliminating vegan and vegetarian products that are processed as well. if you are purchasing these items, read the labels and do your research and make sure that they contain healthy ingredients that also conform to a plant-based diet.

On this diet, aside from animal products, it is important to reduce the amount of sugar and salt that you are consuming. For this reason, most baked goods should be eliminated from your diet. Of course, it may be that you can find baked goods made with whole wheat flour, honey, and a vegan egg product. But this may be another chemical concoction that does not include animal products. If you are making a change in your diet to improve your health, sugar we'll just have to be a casualty a healthy lifestyle.

Avoid eating white carbohydrates. This would include white rice, white bread, and white potatoes. These foods are not converted to energy easily and 10 to cause spikes in sugar levels, causing a release of insulin into your system. As an alternative, make sure to eat whole grains such as brown rice, whole fiber bread, and whole-grain pasta to supplement your diet. These items are processed more easily in your system and allow insulin to be released slowly over time decreasing the spikes that occur with processed carbohydrates. It is simply a fact that healthy lifestyles limit the amount of sugar included in your diet.

In all cases of the food that you're eating, try to avoid seasoning with excess amounts of salt. This is a great time to try out new spices and herbs so that you're adding flavor instead of salt to your food. Excess salt also tends to tell your taste buds. By weaning yourself from your reliance on salt, you may find that food tastes better, and you have a broader range of tasty food at your disposal.

Deep-fried foods are a definite negative on your plant-based diet. Again, with healthy foods as the focus of your diet, deep-fried and fatty foods will be eliminated right off the bat. These foods are high in calories and fat. Fried vegetables are not healthy. The fat used in frying the foods tends to be high in bad cholesterol. This is because these fats can be heated to a higher temperature, which allows for foods to cook without the oil burning. The increase in LDL, or bad cholesterol, leads to heart disease, some cancers, and type 2 diabetes. Consistently eating deep-fried foods can contribute to an early death. Frying a green tomato is a great way to ruin perfectly acceptable food. As an alternative, try using air fryers that utilize hot air to make food crispy without adding excess fat. Oven frying isn't another alternative. In this method, food is baked at a high temperature to create a crispy coating. Deep-fried foods are simply unhealthy and should be avoided.

All the Talk About Water—What Does it Mean?

Water is one of the most necessary parts of any diet plan. The consumption of water will help you condition your body to accept all the other minerals, vitamins, and nutrients that you are consuming regularly. Water is the catalyst for healthy cells and a healthy body. When you consume more than enough water, you store enough in your body to assist in lubricating joints, helping with the circulation of blood throughout your body, delivering vital nutrients two organs throughout your body, and regulating your body temperature. A woman's body is about 55% water. That percentage must be maintained so that your body is working efficiently.

Is Alkaline Water Necessary?

Recently, it has become popular to drink alkaline water. This water does not have any scientific evidence backing the claims that it contributes anything to the internal workings of the human body. There are claims that alkaline water increases the blood flow throughout your system. Studies also suggest that for people with acid reflux, a higher pH value may offset the enzyme pepsin, which causes acid reflux. Other studies suggest that the alkaline properties in the water are neutralized by stomach acid and therefore have no measurable, in fact, on the body. Overall, if you are drinking alkaline water, be sure to limit the amount of alkaline water you consume daily. if too much alkaline water is introduced into your system, you may upset the bacteria in your organs and limit their effectiveness in combating bad bacteria entering your system. Also, excess amounts of alkaline in your system may upset your normal pH level, and your stomach in the process. Overall, most medical research points to the fact that there is no real benefit found in consuming alkaline water. Plain water is sufficient for helping the body to function.

How Much Water Should I Drink?

The easy answer to this question of how much water should one drink each day is 8 cups. That means eight 8 oz glasses of water. The way that women over 50 should drink the water may make a difference. To stave off dehydration, it is suggested that you constantly sip from water throughout the day. This is more effective than downing all the water at once to get it out of the way. You will need more water if the outside temperatures are high if you have a fever, are experiencing vomiting or diarrhea, or if you live and a high-altitude. You can easily accomplish drinking 8-9 cups of water each day if you carry a water bottle with you. Take sips throughout the day even if you're not thirsty. If you feel thirsty, you are probably already becoming dehydrated. Dehydration hurts your body. You may feel fatigued and suffer from mild mood swings. Not consuming enough water also contributes to constipation and kidney stones. Your body needs adequate amounts of water every day to keep it running smoothly.

If you're looking for ways to be sure you're drinking enough water, try adding lemon juice or lime juice to your water. These juices contribute to weight loss and overall health. do not add sugar to your water and avoid sugary drinks and alcohol as well. They added calories and may not provide any beneficial comments to your health. If you're working out, drink more water. You will need to replace the water that you lose through sweat. don't wait until you feel thirsty while you're working out. Keep hydrated throughout your workout and don't have the water you drink at that time in your 8 glasses of water.

Do Smoothies Count as Water?

Smoothies and other beverages count in your total water consumption for a day. It is important to remember not to include sugary beverages and alcohol in your daily count. You can accent your daily intake of water by including some foods with high water content. These include food like watermelon, celery, cucumbers, spinach, and cauliflower. These fruits and vegetables contain fiber and water, which will assist digestive functions well adding to overall health.

Beverages like milk, tea, and coffee are also considered in the count. They add to your overall hydration and may provide nutrients to your body as well. It is best to try to avoid empty calories in the beverages you consume. Beverages like smoothies, without sugar, are a perfect addition to your liquid count because they provide nutrients, fiber, and hydration. You may want to set up a schedule for drinking water so that you remember to stay hydrated throughout the day. with all of the options available, it may seem that drinking 8 cups of water will be easy. It may be easier on some days than others. It's best to set up a routine so that you are sure to drink the minimum amount of water throughout the day

Will I Always Be Running to the Bathroom?

You will experience more frequent trips to the bathroom as you begin to increase your consumption of water. This is not a bad thing. When you drink enough water, your urine will appear pale to clear. This is the best-case scenario for urination. Drinking a lot of water flushes out your kidneys and may prevent kidney stones. This is the benefit of drinking adequate amounts of water. Sometimes you have to plan when you will drink water based on having access to a bathroom. If it is to make these plans, do it. You may also want to drink a preponderance of the water early in the day so that you're not disrupted often while trying to sleep. As your body becomes used to the increased amount of water you're drinking, you will likely can your body on a schedule that suits your needs. Having to go to the bathroom often is annoying, but consider it a slightly negative consequence of improving your overall health and well-being.

Chapter 4: Reset Your Exercise Plan

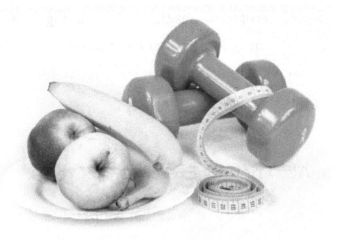

As you surpassed the age of 50, the need for exercise increase. In the past, you may have been exercising to maintain a healthy weight and improvement of cardiovascular health. You were likely concentrating on running or walking in an attempt to increase your heart rate and burn calories. After turning 50, new health issues sneak into your life. There is now also a need for women to offset the loss of muscle mass that tends to show itself as we age. There is also the loss of bone density, and these are physical situations that need to be addressed. Exercises must now incorporate weight training to increase muscle mass and enhance bone growth as well. New exercises must be established if you were not previously doing them so that you can continue to be healthy with adequate mobility as you age. You may need to adjust the type of exercises that you are doing because of limitations resulting from your current physical situation, and the work you put in may just what you need to improve your flexibility muscle control.

Middle-Age Friendly Exercises

As you age, it may become clear that your body is not as flexible and as it once was. One consequence of the aging process is joint pain. Your joints may be experiencing inflammation caused by the breakdown of cartilage separating the bones in your joints. You may find that you feel pain when performing an exercise, and you may want to make some changes to your exercise program so that you can continue to remain active.

The best way to continue to be active as you grow older is to adjust your workouts so that any pain you feel is not debilitating or exacerbated by the exercise process. Beginning an exercise session by warming up and following with a good stretch. Tendons and ligaments are not as flexible as they were when you were younger. You need to prepare your body for exercise, so there is no shot to the system. Speaking of shocking the system, you may find that your workout is a challenge by pounding and changing directions. Because of the lack of flexibility in your joints, sudden changes of direction and stopping and starting can be a painful endeavor. It's time to introduce low impact exercises to your lifestyle if you have not already made the change.

Take time to investigate what types of exercises do uncomfortable doing as you grow older. Activities like swimming, cycling, and walking may need to replace previous activities like jogging and sports like basketball. There is still ample opportunity to participate in athletic endeavors, but they should be activities that highlight smooth transitions of movement and those that do not have a sharp impact on your body.

Participate in exercises that you're comfortable doing. If you can make adjustments to decrease pain and discomfort, oh, make them. It may be necessary to eliminate some physical activity from your lifestyle, but try to replace them with lower impact exercises. Even if you have a sedentary lifestyle, you may still be able to begin working out and increase your levels of activity over time. The important aspect is to get up and move. Use your muscles so that you offset the loss of muscle mass and bone density. This can be done by joining a gym, walking, and or performing exercises in your home. Sometimes, you don't even need to go to the gym to get exercise. completing tasks around your house may be just what you need to get some aerobic exercises under your belt. Raking leaves and mowing the lawn may be good ways to multitask and get some exercise and while completing household chores. Scrubbing floors and walls may not be your favorite way to exercise, but they will get your muscles moving and can get your heart rate up.

If you're just starting to exercise, start slow. You can begin by walking for short periods and then working out to longer periods of activity. Concentrate on sustaining exercise for 10 to 15-minute periods. As you continue to exercise, you'll be able to exercise for longer periods. When you can comfortably walk for 30 minutes, it's time to introduce anaerobic exercises to your regimen.

Embrace Anaerobic Exercise

Over the age of 50, anaerobic exercises are beneficial for women. Anaerobic exercises have periods of strength training I sent by periods of cardio training. Commonly, this is called interval training. Interval training can be done in one session or throughout the week. It's a good idea to complete two and a half hours of aerobic exercise each week. This should be accompanied by an hour and a half of strength training exercises during the week as well. Aerobic exercises are those that increase your heart rates like swimming, dancing, walking, and cycling. Strength training generally consists of exercises using weights that are designed to increase muscle throughout the body. This may take the form of working out with weights or machines but can also be as simple as calisthenics like push-ups and squats. The point is, you don't have to join a gym to work out and exercise. You can join a gym and get a trainer who can assist you in determining the best exercises for your body. On the other hand, you should use items commonly found in your home to reach the same results is going to the gym.

Some anaerobic exercises that you can do at home are push-ups, sit-ups, and Pilates. For many people, it may be as simple as finding an exercise blog on the internet and working out in your living room. The internet may also offer sessions in yoga there you can perform at home. Yoga is a good way to start exercising since it encompasses all the elements I'll exercise that you need. The sustained movement will be good for your cardiovascular system, the movements are designed to build strength eye muscles and bones, and you will be stretching and improving your flexibility. If you can't or don't want to take a class in a gym, search the internet to find a suitable workout online. You and your body will appreciate increase activity and muscle tone.

If You Can't Run, Walk; If You Can't Walk, Ride

Any type of exercise that you are achieving will be beneficial, and building strength and improving your health. You'll find that if you have previously been exercising, you only need to accept your limitations and adjust your workouts accordingly. if you have always been a runner, you may find that your knee joints prohibiting the continuation of that activity. burning knee replacement, you may simply need to switch to swimming instead of driving. You may be able to burn a sufficient number of calories by swimming, and the pressure on your joints is non-existent in the water. This allows you to reduce the pain of your workout.

Working out in a gym or at home on equipment, you may need to switch from a treadmill to an elliptical. The elliptical eases the pressure on the knees and allows you to have a cardio workout without the pounding of your joints. Stationary and recumbent bicycles are also alternatives to running and jogging. These activities provide cycling exercises that increase muscle and cardio strength.

The point is, your workout can be strenuous, without the pressure and pain may have been feeling and previous workouts. The deterioration of the body can be reversed through continued exercises focusing on strength and cardiovascular exertion. Don't stop working out because you are unable to do what you were previously doing. The aging process may require changes to your routine, but it does not have to end your workouts. There's no shame in making adjustments. You may have to change activities, but the change does not have to limit your workout experience. You can get just as much exercise as swimming is running. This is just an example of how you can add new exercises to your old spirit to accommodate your new physical limitations.

Most Exercises Can Be Adapted to Your Level of Fitness and What Your Body Can Withstand

If you have taken a fitness class, you know that instructors offer modifications to many of the movements demonstrated in the class. You may need to make your modifications to exercises and activities that you're used to participating in. this may be necessary due to changes in your physical abilities, or your general fitness level. Because there are often illnesses and health issues that begin to plague us as we move through middle age, it's best to listen to your body and change the exercises and movements to match the current physical abilities. If you are just starting in exercising or a specific activity, you may need to modify the exercise so that it does not create a severe impact on your joints and bones. May also be limited in mobility, and though you will want to press your body into new shapes and movements, you don't want to strain any muscles attendance. Exercise should not be painful, but there may be some discomfort as you push your body to break thresholds and improve.

Again, having a personal trainer is one way to learn modification is two exercises. on the other hand, you still have to listen to your own body and know what your limits are. By knowing what you can comfortably accomplish, you will be able to stretch the current abilities to the next level. Practice and consistency will net improvement in your physical I've been honest.

It's Okay to Take it Slow

Especially if you are just beginning to partake in an exercise program, it will be necessary to go slow. If you reach the age of 50 without a specific exercise routine, introducing one in middle age will take some getting used to. One of the best ways to start exercising is to walk. Begin by walking 3 to 4 days each week for short intervals. Walking is a good all-around exercise and you can improve your fitness levels over time by increasing the time and distance of your walks. You can also add hand-held weights while you walk. This increases your cardiovascular experience and builds muscle. Start with small, light 1lb. weights, then gradually increase the weights up to 3-5 lbs. per hand. When you feel you can, add a new exercise day to your routine. Try to exercise 10-15 minutes per day to start. Increase the length by 5-minute intervals until you are comfortable exercising for extended periods. The basic recommendation is to exercise at moderate intensity for 30 to 50 minutes, 4 or 5 days a week. It may take some time to work up to that level, and once those levels are reached, you may find that you exceed those recommended amounts. For many, exercise is a chore. For others, it is a hobby. Work to achieve specific fitness levels so that you have goals and can quantify your achievements. You will find that as long as you continue to exercise regularly, your strength, endurance, and flexibility will improve.

Determining Your Level of Fitness

There are five different components of fitness. On the surface, most people will judge your fitness level based on body composition. People will look at you and determine whether you are fit or not based on your physical size. This is an inaccurate judgment a physical fitness. In fact, of the five components, many people are fit in some areas and less fit in other areas. It is important to determine your physical fitness level for each factor in developing an exercise plan that will help you to achieve overall fitness.

The first element of physical fitness is aerobic endurance. This measures how long you can sustain aerobic exercise. Measuring your aerobic endurance requires that you take your resting heart rate, RHR, by measuring your heart rate while you are resting. This may be taken right as you wake up. If you count your heartbeats for 10 seconds, * 6 and you have your resting heart rate. This should be compared with the resting heart rate for people of your age and gender. You have determined your resting heart rate, run or jog for 1 mile. This smile should be completed within the recommended time allowed for people of your age and gender. After completing a mile, measure your heart rate. If it is beating faster than your target heart rate, you're not fit in a category of aerobic endurance.

To improve your aerobic endurance level, keep exercising. Performing cardiovascular exercises like walking, dancing, and running, we'll see improvement if you just continue to perform the activity. Your fitness level should increase over time simply through repetition. You want to aim for your target heart rate to be within an acceptable range. You will be able to feel your fitness level improving in your ability to endure an exercise for longer periods

The next measurement of fitness is muscular strength. To measure your muscular strength, determine how much weight you can bench press for one rep. to increase your fitness in muscular strength, workout with weights. If you are unable to join a gym or do not have weights at home, you can increase your muscular endurance by simply doing push-ups at home. Your body weight will provide a challenge, and if you can do a full push-up, repetition will increase your muscular strength as well.

To determine muscular endurance, perform sit-ups for 1 minute using proper form. Count the number of sit-ups performed during the minute and compared to the average for your gender and age. Classes and routines in martial arts Kama Jiu-Jitsu and kickboxing are good ways to increase muscular endurance. This can also be achieved by participating in Pilates classes that feature interval training and strength exercises.

To measure flexibility, you will measure the amount of reach you have by bending over while either sitting or standing and reaching past your toes. You can increase your flexibility with yoga and Pilates. These types of routines increase your strength as well.

The final measurement is Body Composition. Calculate your BMI to determine your fitness for Body Composition. Body composition will be improved or altered through regular exercise and diet. whether you need to increase your BMI or decrease your BMI, exercises can be a key to achieving your fitness goals as they relate to body composition.

As you can see, there are several factors in determining your fitness level. You will want to increase your fitness level in areas where are you don't measure up.

What to Do at Different Fitness Levels

Some exercises are perfect for all fitness levels. They are easy to build upon so that you can start at any level and continually improve. They are also activities where you can improve with repetition and consistency.

Swimming - Swimming is a perfect exercise for all fitness levels. There will always be the ability to improve your stamina and distance. The exercise in water provides you with buoyancy and does not put stress on your joints and bones. Besides swimming itself, water aerobics fits into this category. Swimming is easy on the body and a way to perform aerobic and strength-building exercises.

Walking - all you need is a pair of comfortable shoes to get out and start exercising. Walking is the easiest and most cost-effective way to get exercise and improve your fitness level. You can start by walking around the block and grow to travel long distances. If you work within a few hours of your home, you may want to use walking as a form of commuting as well as exercise. Also, if you have a dog, walking the dog is a good way to exercise both you and your four-legged friend. If you do not have a dog, perhaps there is a neighborhood dog who can use some exercise and you can be just the person to provide it.

Tai chi – this form of exercise is a martial art that features routine movements with smooth transitions and strength building poses. This is a way to build strength while exercising and integrate relaxation into your exercise program. Tai chi features core-strengthening exercises that are useful to women over 50 who may be subject to diminished core strength and lacking balance.

Check with Your Doctor

You want to be sure to check with your doctor before beginning any exercise plan. This is important to determine that your body is ready for exercise and can sustain the stress put on it during the exercise process. It is best to get tests done to determine your heart and joint health. this is not only true for people embarking on an exercise program, but also for people who exercise regularly. Even though you may not feel that you want to visit a doctor, measuring regular occurrence. Getting your doctor's opinion on minor aches and pains can forestall serious health issues in the future. Exercise is a beneficial activity.

Make sure that you're healthy enough to complete the exercise plan you have in mind.

Progress is Progress…Don't Measure Yourself Against Anyone Else

You mustn't measure your progress in improving your fitness levels against someone else. Your fitness plan is your own. It is important to judge your achievement on your plan and not compare it to someone else. Your fitness goals are personal and design for your own body and needs.

After you assess your fitness level, you will design a fitness plan that addresses the needs you have in the various categories of fitness levels. You may need to increase your fitness level in one or all of the categories. Depending on what your levels are currently, and where you want to be in the future, your fitness goals will be personalized to meet your needs as you work through your fitness activities, you will be able to see where you will be able to make good progress, without worrying that your progress may be slower. The pace of your improvement is not important. Getting out and exercising regularly is important. Moving and participating in physical activity is of supreme importance. By completing a list of goals, you will be able to measure your progress and adjust your goals as you feel necessary.

What to Eat Before and After Exercise

No matter what time of day you plan to exercise, you will need the energy to guide you through your exercise routine. This energy can be found by eating foods made from complex carbohydrates, protein, and fat. You can use fruit as a carbohydrate, and almond butter can serve as your protein and fat. You want to eat a small amount of food before your workout. The food is simply a way to get you through a workout of up to an hour. The simple snack should not be larger than a single serving of carbohydrates about the size of your palm. You should eat this for about an hour or 45 minutes before you plan to work out. You will have the energy to get through the workout and you'll be able to burn fat more efficiently and build muscle.

In a plant-based diet, you may want to stick to nut butter and whole-grain bread products. Even avocado toast, can I provide enough energy to get through your workout. Spreading whole-grain toast with and almond butter sprinkling with flaxseed and raisins is a protein-packed snack that would be a good source of energy. By eating 45 minutes before your workout, the energy will still be in reserve to burn off while you are working out. The energy provided to your muscles will also diminish the feelings of fatigue and muscle soreness after your workout is complete.

Within an hour after your workout, you should eat a post-workout snack. If you're looking to build muscle mass, you'll want to eat protein. many people who are looking to build muscle want to consume at least 18 grams of protein after their workout. You also want to include carbohydrates in the snack after your workout. The carbohydrates will provide fuel for your muscles and help them to recover quickly after a workout.

Eat your post-workout snack within an hour of your workout. You may find that it is most effective to eat within 30 minutes of completing your workout. One way to get the protein into your post-workout snack is to drink a soy or almond milk smoothie with kale, fruit, and a protein-packed seed tossed in.

Basically, both before and after you're working out, you want to include carbohydrates in a protein and your snack or meal. The protein and carbohydrates both serve to help build muscle during the workout, and the carbohydrates help to eliminate muscle fatigue during and after will work out session. You should be able to eat whole foods that have enough protein and carbohydrates to sustain your workouts. If you're working out for longer than 90 minutes, you may need more carbohydrates before you working out. By making sure your kind of carbohydrates are whole grain and complex, the energy is released more efficiently over a longer period.

When is the Best Time to Exercise?

The best way to burn fat during a workout is to exercise on an empty stomach. This means working out in the morning before you first eat. If you're not a morning person, it's okay. The time of your workout doesn't matter. the most efficient timing of exercise is whatever time you set aside to do the exercise. It is most efficient for women over 50 to exercise each day. This can be as simple as a daily walk. This walking exercise may not be solely appropriate as a means of weight loss. Exercising for short periods every day provides your muscles with the opportunity to recover without becoming overly fatigued. If you're looking to burn fat, it's best to exercise on an empty stomach. But if you're looking to gain muscle mass, it's better to eat before exercise.

Food Combinations for Energy

By consuming proteins and carbohydrates before and after your workout, you will increase your energy levels. The proteins will be plant-based, perhaps this is an opportunity to snack on a soy product. But adding a whole food carbohydrate, you will be providing your body with energy. The energy in complex carbohydrates, like those found in whole-grain bread, is released over a longer time than the carbohydrates found in processed foods and simple carbohydrates.

Exercise for Weight Loss

Women over 50 will benefit from both strength and weight training as well as cardiovascular exercise. The cardio and weight training will help to lose that is it is burned off in the exercise process. When you target large muscle groups in weight training, you will also burn more fat. As you increase your strength, you also simultaneously be losing fat. Lifting weights or using hand weights well burn calories quickly. Choose weights that tire out your muscles somewhere around the second set of eight repetitions. You will want to do at least three sets. as you continue to work out, you will increase weights and the number of reps to satisfy your workout needs.

Cardio exercises are important and a good source of weight loss in women over 50. You can walk and gradually work your way to jogging. Even if you do not run or jog, walking briskly can be a good way to burn calories and lose weight.

One of the aspects of weight loss that has not been addressed is stress and sleep. It is important to get adequate amounts of sleep when attempting to lose weight. Stress and sleeplessness increase the levels of cortisol in your system. This is an enzyme that is released in the fight or flight mode of your body. When you're under stress, cortisol is released. Unfortunately, cortisol triggers your body to save fat and store it for future use. This is a historical reaction of your body, which was very useful in ancient times. Today, you don't need the fat stores, and stress causes you to consistently gain weight, especially around your stomach. This is especially unhealthy. Abdominal fat tends to increases heart disease.

For this reason, it is important to attempt to relieve stress in your life. Exercise is a good way to do this. You will be able to see the benefits of daily exercise in an increase in the number of hours you are sleeping, and your quality of sleep may improve. This may, in turn, help you to lose weight and improve your heart health.

Chapter 5: Plant-Based Eating Plan

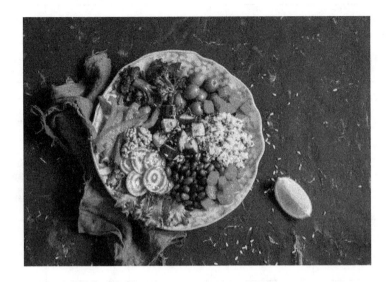

After reviewing all of the pros and cons of switching to a plant-based eating plan, let's take a look at what the actual food plan looks like.

Here is a list of foods that you will want to have on hand in your kitchen to maneuver through a week of recipes on a plant-based diet. These items contain no animal products and can be used to prepare meals for a week.

Proteins	Plant-Based Milk	Fats	Whole Grains	Condiments
Tofu	Coconut Milk,	Olive Oil	Brown Rice	Soy Sauce
Tempeh	Cashew Milk	Coconut Oil	Oats	Vinegar
Edamame	Soy Milk	Grapeseed Oil	Farro	Mustard
	Almond Milk		Quinoa	Nutritional Yeast
	Rice Milk		Whole Grain Pasta	Tahini
	Oat Milk		Barley	

Vegetables	Fruits	Seeds/Nuts	Legumes
Kale	Avocado	Pumpkin Seeds	Peas
Spinach	Berries	Almonds	Chickpeas
Tomatoes	Pears	Cashews	Peanuts
Broccoli	Oranges	Macadamia Nuts	Kidney Beans
Cauliflower	Limes	Natural Peanut Butter	Black Beans
Carrots	Lemons	Almond Butter	Lentils
Peppers	Peaches	Tahini	White Beans
Potatoes	Bananas	Sunflower Seeds	Pigeon Peas
Sweet Potatoes	Cucumbers		
Hard Squash			
Lettuces			

This is a shortlist of the foods you can eat while avoiding animal products. Many fruits and vegetables are best consumed while they are in season. They will have the best flavor and nutrients when they are ripe. You will be able to add a variety of fruits and vegetables to this list throughout the seasons depending on your location. This will allow you to try new things and maybe find a new item that you must have waiting in your pantry.

It is important to avoid certain foods when concentrating on healthy eating. Avoid ready-to-eat meals. The processing involved may include chemicals and preservatives that may not be healthy. This is true for foods you may find on a hot bar in grocery stores. The prepared foods are made outside of your control. If there is a nutritional label and ingredient list, make sure to read it. If it is apparent that the food has been prepared using your standards of whole and natural foods, there should not be any issues.

With the diet restrictions of a plant-based diet, eating whole foods is the best way to consume the vast array of nutrients you expect to find in the limited food selection. Avoid processed sugars and concentrate on natural sugars from fruits for the sugar content of your diet.

Here is a list of foods that are to be avoided if your diet is based on plants.

Fried Foods

Fast Foods

Sugary drinks and treats, including those with artificial sugar

White rice, pasta, bread, and bagels

Processed vegan foods like vegan cheese and vegan sausages and lunch meat.

Frozen dinners

Animal products including meat and dairy products

Some of the foods are unhealthy, like fast food, and others are not rich in nutritional value, like bagels. With the changes to our bodies as we reach the age of 50, it is necessary to minimize unnecessary calories in our diet. Our bodies have a propensity to gain weight. Even with exercise, it is better to eliminate food that will not provide sufficient nutritional value.

Meal Planning

Since you will want to be sure to consume the most nutritious meals possible, make sure to add plenty of color and variety to each meal. The suggested meals are for providing protein and vitamins daily without worrying about calories and fat grams. By eliminating animal products, it is much easier to maintain a healthy calorie count daily. This is, of course, assisted by the lack of refined sugar and fast foods in the new lifestyle. The meal plans can be interchanged and doctored to suit your individual needs. There are snack products that may be added to your daily meal plan. Snacks may consist of raw fruit and vegetables. Roasted edamame and chickpeas are also a nice alternative to chips and pretzels for snacking. They provide a satisfying crunch and have vitamins present in the snack form.

When you are thinking about meal preparations, try to draw on ethnic recipes from countries that have a large vegetarian population. These include many Asian cultures. Using the food they have traditionally eaten as a guideline can help you to find recipes that are satisfying for you and your family as well. You don't have to start from scratch. There are a lot of recipes available that have been pleasing palates for centuries. Foods void of animal proteins do not have to feel incomplete. They are becoming more and more popular. This makes it easy to find foods that are delicious and satisfying. It also makes it more likely that plant-based dairy items will be enriched with vitamins and minerals in manners similar to their animal dairy cousins.

Nutritional yeast is a salt-free seasoning that enhances the flavor of foods like salt. It is a healthier alternative to salt as seasoning. Use salt sparingly. If you do not have any dietary restrictions to salt, it can be used as normal.

	Breakfast	Lunch	Dinner
Monday	Oatmeal made with almond milk, mixed with flax seeds, and topped with blueberries.	Meatless Chilli made with kidney beans, tomatoes, and carrots.	Roasted Vegetable burrito bowl with brown rice, corn, avocado and black bean salsa, lettuce

			and soy milk sour cream.
Tuesday	Smoothie made with coconut milk, frozen blueberries, frozen strawberries, and kale.	Bottomless salad of romaine lettuce, sunflower seeds, pumpkin seeds, cucumber, chopped cabbage, corn, and chickpeas.	Butternut squash noodles seasoned with nutritional yeast and tahini sprinkled with pumpkin seeds.

Wednesday	Plain Almond milk yogurt topped with fruit and unsweetened coconut and walnuts.	Avocado toast. Mash avocado with lime juice. Spread over whole wheat toasted bread and sprinkle with pumpkin seeds	Roasted portobello mushrooms served with blanched green beans and brown rice mixed with corn, red peppers, and soy sauce.
Thursday	Whole grain toast spread with almond butter and topped with sliced banana and sprinkled with raisins.	Soup made from emulsified potatoes, chopped celery, fresh corn kernels, peas, and bell peppers, and	Zucchini noodles topped with tomato sauce made from diced tomatoes cooked with onions, garlic, carrot cubes,

		vegetable stock.	eggplant, and diced firm tofu.
Friday	Smoothie made from soy milk, frozen or fresh mango, berries, and spinach.	Arugula salad with spinach, diced cucumber, red bell pepper, pecans, and tossed in a dressing of natural peanut butter blended with rice wine vinegar and grapeseed oil.	Lentil soup with carrots and kale. The vegetable stock base has lentils and other vegetables added to it.
Saturday	Grits made with water and seasoned with	Cassava and Coconut flour tortillas filled with refried black beans,	Stir-fried vegetables with tofu added. Add vegetables like

	nutritional yeast.	topped with lettuce, tomato, and onion.	sugar snap peas or bamboo shoots, cabbage or bok choy, and carrots. Season with soy sauce and ginger and serve over brown rice.
Sunday	Shredded sweet potatoes, kale, orange bell pepper, onion, cooked in olive oil, and topped with sautéed mushrooms.	Tofu lettuce wraps with water chestnuts and rice noodles. Miso soup with little bits of tofu floating in it.	Vegetable curry with sweet potato cubes, chopped onions, broccoli, carrots, and tofu. Create a sauce with tahini, garlic,

			tomatoes, and curry powder.

If you are accustomed to cooking meals, it may be easiest for you to create your recipes with your current knowledge and the food you have in your home.

To do this, make sure you have foods on hand that will assist you in making a meal without having to run to the store.

Breakfast Staples

Breakfast foods can be some of the easiest to convert to vegan foods. That is if you are determined to limit your breakfast to oatmeal and smoothies. While these items can be set up to be quick and easy in the mornings, other ingredients can be used to make a hot breakfast.

Substitute tofu for eggs. Add potatoes and vegetables to make a hot farm-style breakfast. Add avocado for texture and additional nutritional value. Sauté with spinach or kale, and you have a healthy, protein-filled breakfast.

Keep on Hand

Firm or extra firm tofu

Avocado

Spinach

Kale

Tomato

Potatoes

Oats

Fresh and Frozen Fruits

Grits

Unsweetened Almond Milk

Honey

Buckwheat flour

Baking Powder

Nuts and seeds for texture

Chickpea flour

You may want to keep vegan-friendly tortillas on hand as well. Chickpea flour can be used as a substitute for eggs as well. The chickpea flour allows you to work with a product that is similar in consistency to eggs. Though the flavor may not be exactly like eggs, it is close. If mixed with vegetables and cooked with flavor and seasonings, the skillet breakfast is easily within reach.

If you are planning to serve a hot breakfast that is neither oatmeal nor grits, you may have to re-think your definition of breakfast foods. For many omnivores, breakfast is made up of exactly the foods that are animal-based and animal proteins. Consider a meal of bacon or sausage, eggs, and white toast with butter and possibly jelly. While toast and jelly are plant-based foods, white toast has minimal nutritional value and fiber and is not included in the new meal plan. Jelly is sugary, though you can switch to no-sugar-added fruit spreads. So, it is possible to convert the breakfast full of animal products and foods with sugar and lacking in nutritional value to a delicious and healthy plant-based breakfast.

Chop vegetables to be used in your skillet. This can be an assortment of veggies you have in your refrigerator and pantry. After they have all cooked, prepare to add the "eggs" For the eggs, use chickpea flour and mix with water until it is the consistency of scrambled eggs. Pour over the vegetables and let it heat until set. Chop up to look like eggs. Season with turmeric and nutritional yeast.

This will not taste like the skillet you may be used to eating, but that's okay. Consider your new diet and lifestyle, an adventure that will introduce you to new flavor palates and expand your imagination to how food can taste and be satisfying. Most of the foods you will want to keep on hand are available in most grocery stores. Plant-based diets have become so commonplace that general stores have a section of vegan and vegetarian foods. Though soy products are available in the form of vegan sausages and vegan egg products made from beans, read labels carefully to determine that the foods are whole foods, and meet your standards. Read labels and look up any items on the list that you are not clear on the definition.

Oatmeal and smoothies are common breakfast staples for many people. Make sure you have plenty of produce on hand to add to smoothies, with fruits and nuts for the toppings of the oatmeal. You may use any plant-based milk product to make oatmeal. The toppings of fresh fruit, coconut, and nuts will make a satisfying breakfast. Add chia or flaxseed to add protein to the oatmeal. You can also add nut jars of butter to the oatmeal while it is hot for flavor and additional nutrients.

Lunch Staples

Lunch can be a good opportunity for light food with a lot of flavors. This is often where you will find soups and salads in your menu repertoire. When you are planning your lunch meals, you may be able to utilize leftovers from a previous meal. This is especially true if you are making soups and/or salads for your lunch. Because you will want to have a wide variety of foods and flavors, it is a good idea to have items in your pantry that are specific for making soups and salads.

Keep on Hand

Vegetable Stock

Quinoa

Grape Tomatoes

Avocado

Spelt Bread

Whole Grain Bread

Whole Grain Pita

Fresh Vegetables for raw or roasting

Hummus

Red Peppers

Baby Spinach

Arugula

As far as soups go, you will want to have a soup base available for you. This may come in the form of an organic prepared vegetable broth or stock. You may also find that you want to make your vegetable stock. You can keep your stock in the freezer or, if you like, the stock can be scanned and kept in your pantry. If you have fresh and frozen vegetables on hand, making soup is quick and easy. You may be able to use recipes that you have used in the past and adapt them to plant-based friendly recipes. Instead of proteins from animals, you can use vegetable proteins like beans or tofu. It may make for interesting flavor combinations to simply add additional vegetables instead of an animal protein to your soup.

Instead of using dairy as a base for cream soups, you can use white potatoes as a thickener for soup. Run the cooked potatoes through an immersion blender while they are in hot vegetable stock or water.

This will create a nice thick base for your soup, but it will not be as creamy. If you want a creamy soup, you will probably want to add coconut milk or cashew milk. The coconut milk can be easily found as an affordable cream substitute. Cashew milk is more difficult to track down. When you use coconut milk, you end up with that coconut tropical flavor. If a milky consistency is not required, that is when you may want to use potatoes.

Aside from potatoes, you can also use leeks to create a creamy consistency for your soup. Leeks create a nice oniony flavor that you can build upon to make a nice soup for lunch or dinner. If you have flavors like ginger carrots, you may invent a delicious meal by using your imagination and whatever is on hand in your pantry and the refrigerator. Remember that you always want to add an abundance of ingredients to all your meals. This is how you'll be sure to get all the nutrition recommended daily. Keep a variety of foods available to you, and you'll be able to serve them and use them for cooking.

If you do not require a hot meal for lunch, you can put together a meal out of odds and ends in your refrigerator. This may include crackers, fruits, vegetables, and easy sandwiches made with the vegetables and avocado or hummus. You can also put together a tabbouleh salad or a salad made with quinoa and vegetables. Use anything on the condiment list to bind together the vegetables in the salad. Serving these items with spelled bread, pita, or whole fiber bread will make a lunch that's easily put together and ready to take on the go. By lunchtime, you are around halfway through your day, and you should have consumed about half of the water you need to drink during the day. If you're packing breakfast and lunch, make sure you have the opportunity to drink water before during, and after your meals.

Dinner Staples

Dinner is often a big meal involving partners, friends, and family. Use the opportunity to be creative and provide a variety of foods in a delicious medley of foods. The key is to make food where the animal protein is not missed by people who eat meat. You may even want to feel like you are eating meat if you are changing to a plant-based diet strictly for health purposes.

Keep on Hand

Extra Firm Tofu

Vegan Tortillas

Broccoli

Bok Choy

Carrots

Almonds

Walnuts

Brown Rice

Whole Grain Pasta

Spiral Cut Zucchini

Soy Sauce

Tempeh

Legumes

Lentils

Spinach

Kale

Since dinner will probably be your largest meal of the day, you will want it to be filing and full of nutrition. You can use portobello mushrooms as a serving that has the texture and size of meat. Though this may seem to lack in originality, you will have an opportunity to season the mushroom and inventive ways. You also have to serve side dishes that may be primarily made up of vegetables. You can use the whole wheat pasta and brown rice to provide an accent to vegetables that you are using to serve with the portobello mushrooms. As far as flavor profiles, you will want to find and develop recipes that utilize vegetables available to you in your area during the seasons that they are available. This is a good opportunity to use spices and herbs to jazz up your meals. Use sauces to create delicious stir-fries, and you can adapt recipes like your favorite spaghetti sauce and add to spiral cut zucchini or to top whole-grain pasta. These kinds of pasta are readily available and made from chickpeas and whole wheat. They are thought to be considerably healthier than white flour pasta.

Making a flavorful sauce will go a long way toward making a satisfying meal. Add as many ingredients as you are comfortable using. If you are staying away from carbohydrates and sugar, you should feel comfortable by eating as much as you like. unlike some other high-protein diets, the elimination of animal products reduces the fat that he will likely be consumed regularly. Be sure not to exceed your calorie count for the day. Also, keep a tally of the nutritional value of a food that you're eating so that you are sure so have enough of each nutritional element in your diet. You may find that you need to take vitamin supplements. Try to make these adjustments through your diet, but if it isn't happening, it's better to take a supplement then do without.

Snack Staples

Snacks are important. You don't want to end up cheating on your diet plan because you did not feel satisfied. Luckily, there are many plant-based snack items that you can find on the grocery shelves. These include chips made from root vegetables like beets, turnips, and sweet potatoes. They're often organic and lightly salted. You can also trust in yourself and make your snacks like edamame and chickpeas. You can roast these items, season them with spices and herbs, and create a new specialty item straight for your kitchen.

Whole fruits are a good way to snack, especially if you are looking for dessert. An apple or an orange may be the perfect addition to your meal plan. Berries and tropical fruits will also satisfy your sweet tooth with their natural sugars. On a plant-based diet, you can eat as many fruits as you like. This is a great advantage over a low-carb diet. By switching to plant-based foods, many high-calorie foods are eliminated from your diet. It is a good opportunity to enjoy the bounty of nature.

Creating meals on a plant-based diet is not as difficult as it may seem. If you are not accustomed to preparing your meals, it may be a challenge. On the other hand, if you are used to cooking, or someone in your household typically cooks, it is not difficult to adapt tried-and-true recipes to fit into a plant-based meal plan. The most difficult part of planning meals is making sure there are significant nutrients involved in each meal. Because we are used to consuming animal proteins, it's necessary to find proteins and calcium that the body can use to provide strength and energy. Also, make sure you are eating enough iron to stave off iron deficiencies.

Make it a priority to read labels and learn about the foods that you are planning to eat. Switching to a plant-based diet is a learning process, but the rewards are great. You will find that your health can improve, you can lose weight, and many of the small ailments like skin issues and minor aches and pains made evaporate.

There will be plenty of opportunities in grocery stores to purchase plant-based foods that are not healthy. If you are considering that your plant-based diet is vegan, several food options fit this criterion. These include snack chips, cookies, sugary beverages, and soda. These things need to be removed from your kitchens and pantries. The mindset that you can eat all plant-based items must be avoided. Use good judgment in what you eat. If you are adopting this meal plan to improve your health and prospects for a healthy life, do not sabotage yourself by purchasing and consuming foods that don't fit into a healthy meal plan. you may find that you are most successful on this meal plan if you do plan each meal and snack during your day. This can make for a very successful change in lifestyle as you always have food available, and you will be eating at the prescribed times, foods that are perfectly allowable on your plan. Incorporating exercise into your lifestyle will assist you in creating a healthier body. Drink lots of water to be sure you are flushing out toxins from your system and keeping your system hydrated. Hydration is important to maintaining the development of cells in your body.

A lot of ways these plant-based meals make sense. Our lifestyles are completely different from the lifestyles of our carnivorous ancestors who came before us. We are no longer hunters and gatherers. Our food comes packaged and ready to cook. We go to the gym to get the exercise that our families before we got by tending their farms and families. By paring down the amount of food we eat and planning meals that avoid animal meat and dairy products, we are taking steps to improve overall health and wellness in our aging bodies. For women over 50, there are many changes and adjustments to be made to lifestyle, diet, and health. Using the meal plans from above as examples, you can construct a sustainable diet plant that uses everyday items found in most grocers. The meal plans offer suggestions on how to construct recipes that use vegetables and whole grains to fill empty stomachs while avoiding animal products. Use the pantry items as a baseline to fill your shelves with items you may want to keep on hand to be able to easily make meals that you and your family will appreciate.

Conclusion

Thank you for making it through to the end of *Diet and Exercise for Women Over 50*, let's hope it was informative and able to provide you with all of the tools you need to achieve your goals in weight loss and a healthier lifestyle.

As women grow older, there are a variety of changes occurring within their bodies. Having a great deal of impact, the reduction of estrogen often causes weight gain and a slower metabolism. A plant-based diet, with adjustments for the particular requirements of women over fifty years old, is a wonderful way to lose weight while relieving some of the aches and pains experienced as the lack of estrogen takes hold. By adapting to a diet that is rich in nutrients and vitamins, you will be able to maintain a healthy lifestyle and eschew meat at the same time. Animal proteins are not necessary for healthy living.

To be successful with any change to your diet, it is best to record what you are eating and how your body reacts to the food and exercise that you are utilizing. As you work to maintain a record of your lifestyle, you may catch yourself reverting to old habits and when you are feeling a certain way or spending time with a group of people. Family members can be the most effective form of sabotage. Be armed with your records and journals to combat against failing to remain motivated. There is nothing like past success to motivate you towards new successes. Make sure you eat lots of vegetable fiber and drink lots of water. Count calories to be sure you are consuming enough calories, and not too many calories. The path a healthy body is outlined in the book. Take on the challenge of healthy living, and you will be feeling strong in no time.

You have the tools to be successful in losing weight and building bone and muscle. Follow the plant-based meal plans as an outline for the life you want to live.

Finally, if you found this book useful in any way, a review on Amazon is always appreciated!

CPSIA information can be obtained
at www.ICGtesting.com
Printed in the USA
LVHW080118171020
668893LV00004B/488